CRITICAL THINKING
CASES IN RESPIRATORY CARE

CRITICAL THINKING
CASES IN RESPIRATORY CARE

Kathleen J. Wood, MED, RRT
Associate Professor of Respiratory Care
Director of Clinical Education
Respiratory Care Department
Massasoit Community College
Brockton, Massachusetts

 F. A. DAVIS COMPANY • Philadelphia

F. A. Davis Company
1915 Arch Street
Philadelphia, PA 19103

Printed in the United States of America

Last digit indicates print number: 10 9 8 7 6 5 4 3

Publisher, Health Professions: Jean-François Vilain
Senior Editor: Lynn Borders Caldwell
Developmental Editor: Crystal Spraggins
Cover Designer: Louis J. Forgione

As new scientific information becomes available through basic and clinical research, recommended treatments and drug therapies undergo changes. The author and publisher have done everything possible to make this book accurate, up to date, and in accord with accepted standards at the time of publication. The author, editors, and publisher are not responsible for errors or omissions or for consequences from application of the book, and make no warranty, expressed or implied, in regard to the contents of the book. Any practice described in this book should be applied by the reader in accordance with professional standards of care used in regard to the unique circumstances that may apply in each situation. The reader is advised always to check product information (package inserts) for changes and new information regarding dose and contraindications before administering any drug. Caution is especially urged when using new or infrequently ordered drugs.

Library of Congress Cataloging-in-Publication Data

Wood, Kathleen J., 1959–
    Critical thinking : cases in respiratory care / Kathleen J. Wood.
        p.   cm.
    Includes bibliographical references and index.
    ISBN 0-8036-0153-0 (alk. paper)
    1. Respiratory therapy—Case studies. 2. Critical thinking.
3. Medical logic. I. Title.
    [DNLM: 1. Respiratory Therapy—methods. 2. Respiratory Therapy—
case studies. 3. Decision Making. WB 342 W876c 1998]
RC735.I5W66 1998
616.2′0046—dc21
DNLM/DLC
for Library of Congress   97-10615

Foreword

The respiratory care profession has changed dramatically over the past 35 years. Initially, those who provided assistance to physicians during the treatment of patients with pulmonary disease were asked to think very little. Moving equipment from one patient to another and following the doctor's orders were the primary duties of respiratory care practitioners (RCPs) in the early years. Today, however, RCPs are called on to help evaluate patients and to determine the appropriate treatment plan. The ideal RCP not only carries out the plan but also evaluates the results and makes timely suggestions to the attending physician for change during the patient's hospital course. Today, the competent RCP is an extension of the eyes and ears of the physician.

The cognitive skill of critical thinking is the cornerstone of modern patient care by RCPs. Without critical thinking skills, practitioners are not likely to administer appropriate care or make timely suggestions for changing the care plan. This deficiency leads to a number of problems, with inadequate and dangerous patient care at the top of the list. Respect from other health care providers and growth of the profession depend on the ability of RCPs to apply critical thinking to their jobs.

Educators in the health professions have recognized for many years the need for critical thinking among clinicians but often have done very little to act on the deficiency within their own students. A number of excuses are offered, but the results are the same: Graduates either learn to think critically on their own during the initial years of practice and succeed, or they spend many years floundering as clinicians. In either case, educators do a disservice to their students and the patients they serve when they do little or nothing to promote critical thinking in their students.

Fortunately, help has arrived. Kathleen Wood has written a text to help students and clinicians analyze information, think critically about the data, and make sound decisions based on an investigation of the facts. Now respiratory care students can more rapidly develop the important cognitive skill of critical thinking by reviewing the case examples in this text. The case studies cover a wide range of topics, from common problems such as asthma to more challenging dilemmas with multiple trauma. Intermittently provided throughout the cases are questions called "Thought Prompts," which direct the reader to ponder key issues related to the situation. These questions represent the crucial matter of each chapter because they encourage the reader to engage in the cognitive activities that promote critical thinking and optimal patient care. The readers of this text must consider each question carefully to gain the most benefit from reviewing the case studies.

Respiratory care students in the second year of their program and practicing clinicians will benefit greatly from studying this text and responding to the Thought Prompts. By the time the reader completes several chapters, he or she should be well on the way to thinking more critically and developing the cognitive skills so important to the care of patients with cardiopulmonary disease. The more quickly we move away from having our students memorize lists and regurgitate facts and move toward critical thinking, the better off our patients will be.

Robert L. Wilkins, PhD, RRT
Chairman and Professor
Department of Cardiopulmonary Sciences
School of Allied Health Professions
Loma Linda University
Loma Linda, California

Preface

The importance of critical thinking to the profession of respiratory therapy cannot be overemphasized. Simply put, respiratory care practitioners (RCPs) with the ability to think critically are better and more valued professionals. Students with good general critical thinking abilities make better students, and at least one study suggests that these students may even perform better on the information gathering (IG) section of the NBRC Clinical Simulation Examination.[1]

In addition, the ability to write good respiratory care plans, particularly in the nonacute settings, is yet another valuable skill for RCPs. *Critical Thinking: Cases in Respiratory Care* will help students and RCPs focus on the development of the skills essential to this planning process.

The book features a problem-based approach to learning, which promotes concentration on attacking problems with solid critical thinking ability. Critical thinking skills include interpretation, analysis, inference, explanation, evaluation, and self-regulation. Stimulating learning activities and exercises that promote development of these skills are included in the book. In addition, the AARC Clinical Practice Guidelines are used as a primary reference for all applicable clinical situations.

The text provides an opportunity for students to interact with clinical situations in a safe learning environment rather than in actual practice. This "think before you leap" approach provides students with a sound foundation for the application of critical thinking concepts. After all, problem solving, which results from transferring previously learned information to a current situation, occurs when the learning is supported by multiple and various opportunities for practice. The cases in this book provide such practice opportunities while minimizing the stressors of actual practice. Thus, concepts and approaches learned well under optimal learning conditions may be transferred more completely and readily to true clinical practice conditions.

The text is organized in a developmental sequence, beginning with descriptions of critical thinking, problem-based learning, assessment, development of care plans, time management, and evaluation of process and outcome. The major component of the book—the cases—follows. These cases progress in difficulty as the book proceeds. The first case focuses on primary knowledge of respiratory care, whereas subsequent cases involve increasingly more complex issues. Each case is presented as a medical record consisting of a scenario, flow charts, diagnostic lists, critical daily notations, and summaries. "Concept maps" representing the entire case are also included.

Cases are interspersed with questions called "Thought Prompts," which allow the student an opportunity for inquiry and interaction. The interactions may be with peers or tutors, may involve group discussions, or may involve consultation with other resources, inside or outside of the classroom. The student's active participation is advised at these junctures.

Each chapter ends with review questions, which allow students to test their knowledge of the material just presented. Answers to the questions appear at the back of the book.

Critical Thinking: Cases in Respiratory Care is a tool to help students learn how to think critically, thereby preparing them for the Clinical Simulation Examination as well as the real world. Department managers can also use the text to sharpen their employees' critical thinking and protocol skills.

Enjoy!

KW

---

1. Shelledy, DC et al: Effects of content, process, computer-assisted instruction, and critical thinking ability on students' performance on written clinical simulations. Respiratory Care Education Annual 6:11–30, 1997.

The author and the publisher wish to acknowledge the following educators who carefully reviewed the manuscript for this book:

Lawrence A. Dahl, EdD, RRT
Instructor/Program Director
Respiratory Therapy Program
Hawkeye Community College
Waterloo, Iowa

William F. Galvin, MSEd, RRT, CPFT
Assistant Professor
School of Allied Health
Program Director
Respiratory Care Program
Gwynedd Mercy College
Sumneytown Pike
Gwynedd Valley, Pennsylvania

Pamela Griffin, RRT, BSN, MEd
Program Director
Department of Respiratory Therapy
Thomas Technical Institute
Thomasville, Georgia

Stanley M. Pearson, MSEd, RRT, C-CPT
Program Coordinator
Department of Health Care Professions/Respiratory Care
Southern Illinois University at Carbondale
College of Applied Sciences and Arts
Carbondale, Illinois

Robert L. Wilkins, PhD, RRT
Chairman and Professor
Department of Cardiopulmonary Sciences
School of Allied Health Professions
Loma Linda University
Loma Linda, California

Contents

1 | An Introduction to Problem-Based Learning

Learning Objectives

After reading the chapter and performing the activities within it, the learner will be able to:

- Define and elaborate on the concept of problem-based learning (PBL).
- Apply the concept of PBL to the discipline of respiratory care (RC).
- Apply PBL as a learning strategy in improving RC practice and national board performance.
- State supporting and opposing arguments concerning PBL.

Key Words and Phrases

Cause-and-effect diagramming
Collaboration
Concept mapping
Critical thinking
Decision making

Information gathering
Integration
Outcomes
Problem-based learning (PBL)
Recall, analysis, and application

DEFINING ELEMENTS OF PROBLEM-BASED LEARNING

If knowledge is an acquired state, then learning must be an active process. For learning to be active, the learner needs involvement with the subject that is to be understood. This active status of learning requires motivation, interest, and some sense of the direction the process is taking. Stimulating factors must drive the process. Such factors are found when learners are enabled to perform in problem-solving situations. In such an environment they can question and probe areas of the subject under study to gain understanding of the problem and its parts as well as its solution.

The stimulation evoked from such situations is part of the essence of problem-based learning. When we are allowed to actively solve dilemmas by involving ourselves in the inquiry, we gain knowledge and experience at the same time.

Problem-based learning, or *PBL*, consists of the presentation of an "ill-structured problem" to the learner, followed by a guided investigation. This investigation may be conducted through discussion groups, resource searches, tutorial sessions, physical inspections, computer simulations, debates, and other analytic or inquisitive activities.[1] However, the problem under investigation is the core of PBL. The study problem captures the learner's interest and directs the initial formation of perspectives. This process fosters problem solving, information gathering, and decision making.

PBL environments are various and abundant. The spectrum of PBL usage spans from entire courses surrounding one problem to the use of short case problems incorporated into individual classes.[2] The case problems in this book may be considered such supplemental material. They may be used as foundational elements of a course or as added resources for respiratory care (RC) practice. The primary objective of this book is to provide a structural basis for learning and integrating RC material in conjunction with sound critical thinking.

Working within a PBL framework allows the learner to have greater freedom in molding the experience. This is evidenced by the transformation of "lecture halls into discussion forums, where everyone actively engages in the learning."[3] The PBL experience promotes independent learning through its adventure in problem solving. Students are encouraged to seek information using multiple and varied resources.

PROBLEM-BASED LEARNING AND RESPIRATORY CARE

Currently, PBL is the basic curricular component of numerous medical schools. It is quickly becoming the curriculum focus for countless other educational institutions, from elementary schools to postgraduate universities. For example, Aspy[4] describes the positive results garnered by PBL curricula at McMaster University, the University of Mexico, and Harvard-Radcliffe University. Edmondson[5] details the development and success of the PBL program at the College of Veterinary Medicine at Cornell University. Ostwald[6] cites that, at the University of Newcastle, New South Wales, Australia, students are "extremely positive about their PBL experience." He also reports that students have more internal goal orientation, as opposed to students in traditional programs. Stepien[7] reflects on the Illinois Mathematics and Science Academy programs, in which students in grades K through 12 gain skill in "assessment, questioning, information gathering and *collaborating* on the evaluation of hypotheses." And Mishoe[8] illustrates the reorganization of a theoretical curriculum in RC, which would be focused on problems as opposed to content categories.

PBL holds particular promise for allied health education because these students must acquire basic science knowledge as well as technical skill. It is in this arena of technological changes and updates that PBL serves the learner most effectively. In considering RC we must face the fact that no learner can achieve competence in all areas at the novice stage of education. New developments pose challenges for experts as well. Therefore, it is essential to equip learners with the skills that will enable them to continuously acquire and update their proficiency. The emphasis on self-directed learning in PBL enforces the learning of these skills.

ENHANCEMENT OF CRITICAL THINKING

The enhancement of *critical thinking* is the primary outcome of PBL. The problem-solving expeditions within the PBL environment give the learner needed practice and reinforcement in the realm of decision making. If the outcome of one's studies is to make informed judgments, as in RC, then a sanctioned time and place must exist for acquiring the knowledge, attitudes, and behaviors required for such an important mission. By allowing learners to focus on a problem, examine the many facets associated with it, and form judgments and inferences about it, PBL provides such an environment. All of this "thinking work" may be accomplished with the learner in a safe and supportive learning environment.

PROBLEM-BASED LEARNING AND THE NATIONAL BOARD FOR RESPIRATORY CARE EXAMINATIONS

The core elements of performance on the National Board for Respiratory Care (NBRC) written examinations are *recall, analysis, and application* of essential data. It is clear that PBL is closely related to the achievement of competence in these areas. Through active participation in solving a medical problem, learners experience the vast array of interrelationships involved in the problem. For instance, consider the case of a simple pneumonia. There is, of course, the disease entity to recall. This is then related to certain assessments that require analysis to determine the significance of the problem. Then these data undergo *integration* and are often explained. Finally, they are used as a base for care planning. The interrelationship between the "thinking" and "applying" of RC is illustrated in Figure 1–1.

Through the use of PBL programs of study, learners are able to view multiple events occurring simultaneously. This holis-

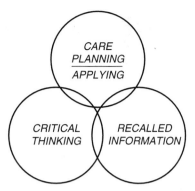

Figure 1–1. Concept map of the interrelationships within the respiratory care (RC) process.

tic approach enables us to easily relate interventions to *outcomes.* For example, a respiratory care practitioner (RCP) uses various methods to enhance patient health, while at the same time he or she forms assumptions about the patient's response. This ability to form reasonable expectations allows practitioners to make sound judgments during the course of treatment. Facing medical problems from an investigative stance, as opposed to a task-oriented position, permits learners the benefit of uncovering important components of a problem and then relating these parts to each other as well as to the desired end result or outcome. Thus the learning process is enhanced. This type of learning promotes the major skills of *information gathering* and *decision making,* the two central categories measured in the NBRC Clinical Simulation Examination (CSE). Working through the case study format in this book allows particular practice in modifying the therapeutic plan, a content area in the CSE.

Tackling problems in a controlled learning environment gives RCPs and students alike the opportunity to practice both information collection and decision making in a supportive and safe atmosphere. PBL presents a very suitable environment for initial learning of concepts with great opportunity for gradual development of understanding and application.

TOOLS FOR ILLUSTRATING CONCEPTS

There are numerous tools for visually displaying concepts. These tools help educators and learners alike. Often a very complex concept may be broken down and revealed more concretely through a drawing of its parts. One tool used throughout this book is concept mapping. *Concept mapping* is the outlining or diagramming of an idea to reveal the relationships among its parts. This type of illustration promotes analytic skill by providing a concrete image of an abstract thought. The visual outline helps in sorting the many parts of complex issues. See Figure 1–2 for a concept map of PBL.

Just as concept mapping aids in the visual outlining of a particular idea, with emphasis on the relationships among its parts, another useful tool, *cause-and-effect diagramming,* aids in illustrating the causal relationships within concepts. Cause-and-effect diagrams provide a more linear outline of an idea.

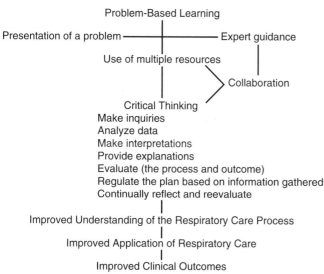

Figure 1–2. Concept map of problem-based learning.

For an example of a cause-and-effect diagram featuring the concept of PBL, see Figure 1–3.

ARGUMENTS FOR AND AGAINST PROBLEM-BASED LEARNING

PBL promotes greater student participation in the learning process and, in so doing, stimulates higher motivation and better retention. Students learning within a PBL environment exceed their traditionally trained peers in integrating basic science knowledge with clinical practice.[9] It is also believed that PBL facilitates lifelong learning.[10]

The benefits are obvious. PBL is an interdisciplinary model of learning, and the present-day practice of medicine is an interdisciplinary arena. The PBL approach brings relevance to learned concepts while promoting the student's ability to solve problems. Its primary outcome is the integration of clinical practice with basic knowledge. Data indicate that learners involved in PBL curricula are mastering essential content within their studies while enjoying the stimulation and integration of learning and relating to the "big picture."[11] Collectively these many advantages of PBL create an opportunity for educators and learners alike to enhance the development of basic knowledge into more advanced practices.

Detractors of PBL cite as its disadvantage the lack of avail-

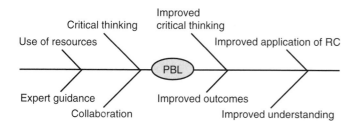

Figure 1–3. Cause-and-effect diagram of problem-based learning.

able data supporting it in the basic sciences. However, Aspy[12] states that medical students involved in PBL courses are better able to integrate their learning and thus transfer more from the basic sciences to their clinical practice situations. Other opponents charge that PBL is merely a fad and has no real impact on learning. Last, and perhaps least, is the notion that educators who already have classes prepared may in fact reject PBL because of resistance or fear.

Summary

This chapter focuses on the concept of PBL as a tool for enabling learning within the discipline of RC. PBL's defining characteristics include the presentation of an ill-structured problem accompanied by guided inquiry into the problem. The use of long or short case studies is discussed as one method for PBL teaching. The application of PBL in preparing learners for credentialing examinations is supported. Some successful PBL experiences are noted as well as the tools of mapping and diagramming ideas. Several supporting and detracting arguments are presented regarding the use of PBL. The reader is urged to see the chapter's reference section for further information on the subject of PBL.

References

1. Stepien, W and Gallagher, S: Problem-based learning: As authentic as it gets. Educational Leadership, April, 1993, pp. 25–28.
2. Ibid, p. 27.
3. Aspy, N, Aspy, C and Quinby, P: What doctors can teach teachers about problem-based learning. Educational Leadership, April, 1993, p. 22.
4. Ibid, pp. 22–23.
5. Edmondson, K: Concept mapping for the development of medical curricula. ERIC Document Reproduction Service No ED 360 322, Atlanta, 1993.
6. Ostwald, MJ, Chen, SE, Varnum, B and McGeorge, D: The application of problem-based learning to distance education. ERIC Document Reproduction Service No ED 359 398, Newcastle, NSW, Australia, 1993.
7. Stepien et al, op cit, p. 25.
8. Mishoe, S: Critical thinking, education preparation and development of respiratory care practitioners. The AARC Distinguished Papers Monograph 2:29–43, 1993.
9. Aspy et al, op cit, p. 24.
10. Kaufman, A et al: The New Mexico experiment: Educational innovation and institutional change. Acad Med 64:285–294.
11. Aspy et al, op cit, p. 24.
12. Ibid.

PRACTICE QUESTIONS

1. PBL may be:
   I. Found in high schools
   II. Practiced in universities
   III. Effective for practical application of learning
   IV. Based on ill-structured problems

   A. I, II, and III
   B. I, II, and IV
   C. II, III, and IV
   D. I and IV
   E. I, II, III, and IV

2. All of the following describe the tool of concept mapping except:
   A. It reveals cause-and-effect data.
   B. It illustrates interrelationship between parts of an idea.
   C. More than one map may be created for a topic.
   D. It provides visual aids for learning a concept.

3. Essential PBL components include:
   I. An ill-structured problem
   II. Structured lecture sessions
   III. Guided inquiry into a problem
   IV. Use of multiple resources by learners
      A. I and II
      B. I, III, and IV
      C. I, II, and III
      D. I, II, and IV
      E. I, II, III, and IV

4. One drawback of PBL may be:
   A. The multidisciplinary nature of a subject
   B. The lack of data proving that PBL enhances basic science knowledge
   C. The need to transfer learned information from theory to practice
   D. Increased student participation
   E. The use of case studies

5. All of the following describe critical thinking except:
   A. Inference making
   B. Analyzing
   C. Recalling information
   D. Evaluating
   E. Interpreting

6. Outcomes of PBL include all of the following except:
   A. Promotion of lifelong learning
   B. Integration of multiple studies
   C. Faster retention of learned material
   D. Facilitation of critical thinking skills
   E. Independent learning

7. Which of the following represent the basic categories found on the NBRC written examinations?
   A. Analysis, synthesis, and argument
   B. Application, translation, and calculation
   C. Problem solving, reasoning, and judgment foundation
   D. Recall, application, and analysis
   E. Probing, solving, and understanding

8. Student participation in PBL programs is:
   A. Increased as compared to traditional settings
   B. A desirable outcome
   C. Encouraged by instructors in PBL
   D. A central goal
   E. All of the above

9. Cause-and-effect diagrams reveal:
   A. Conceptual relationships
   B. Assessment data only
   C. Etiological data only
   D. Causal relationships
   E. Historical data only

10. PBL classes would most likely include:
   I. Group discussions
   II. Guided inquiry into a problem
   III. Independent study
   IV. Memory matrix diagramming
   V. Sequenced instructions for problem solving
      A. I, II, and III
      B. I, III, and V
      C. II and IV
      D. I, II, III, and IV
      E. I, II, III, IV, and V

2 | Critical Thinking in Respiratory Care

Learning Objectives

After reading the chapter and performing the activities within it, the learner will be able to:

- Define critical thinking (CT).
- Identify the skills and subskills of CT.
- List the characteristics of the critical thinker.
- Relate the concept of CT to its use in RC.
- Identify ways to practice and assess CT skills.
- Recognize that the National Board for Respiratory Care (NBRC) assesses CT via its credentialing examination.
- Identify roadblocks to development of sound CT skills.
- Compare and contrast the expert versus novice approach to RC practice and relate this to the level of CT skill.

Key Words and Phrases

Analysis	Inference
Conceptualizations	Interpretation
Contexts	Methods
Criteria	NBRC content areas
Critical thinking (CT)	Ordinary versus critical thinking
Dispositions	Pitfalls and roadblocks
Evaluation	Problem-based learning (PBL)
Evidence	Self-regulation
Expert versus novice thinking	Self-regulatory judgment
Explanation	Structured controversy

CRITICAL THINKING DEFINED

Critical thinking (CT) has gained great attention in all aspects of education. It is not a newly invented type of thinking, but rather an ancient method of thought process. The national attention to CT stems from a basic need to develop a competent workforce capable of adapting to rapidly changing environments. Solid CT skills will enable workers to become proficient in complex tasks. RCPs must deal with complexity, rapid change, and a demand for quick yet correct decision making. CT is the thought process required in such an environment.

Critical thinking is defined as "the process of purposeful, *self-regulatory judgment*. This process gives reasoned consideration to *evidence, contexts, conceptualizations, methods* and *criteria*."[1] Careful, rational, content-specific thinking is a catalyst for self-correction. This type of thinking is based on reason and is supported by *evidence*.

The cognitive skills associated with CT are *interpretation, analysis, evaluation, inference, explanation,* and *self-regulation*.[2] These skills are closely related to the components of the scientific method. The skill differentiating CT from all other cognitive processes is self-regulation. Self-regulation is also most essential to RC practice. This ability permits the practitioner to competently, efficiently, and promptly adapt to changes in clinical practice. Self-regulation also ensures the continuous monitoring and modifying of our practice. These are keys to quality improvement as well.

Each of the cognitive skills is further divided into subskills (Table 2–1). This last grouping represents a most complete list of criteria for defining the mechanisms involved in CT.

Note that CT is not limited to a particular dimension of time. It occurs in the present, is reflective of the past, and is mindful of the future. This dimension of CT has prompted a great many people to refer to the critical thinker as a "reflective thinker." The ideal critical thinker is: habitually inquisitive, well-informed, trustful of reason, open-minded, flexible, fair-minded in evaluation, honest in facing personal biases, prudent in making judgments, willing to reconsider, clear about issues, orderly in complex matters, diligent in seeking relevant information, reasonable in the selection of criteria, focused in inquiry, and

Table 2–1 CRITICAL THINKING SKILLS AND SUBSKILLS

Interpretation
- Categorizing
- Decoding
- Clarifying meaning

Analysis
- Examining ideas
- Identifying arguments
- Analyzing arguments and evidence

Evaluation
- Assessing claims
- Assessing arguments

Inference
- Querying evidence
- Conjecturing alternatives
- Drawing conclusions

Explanation
- Stating results
- Justifying procedures
- Presenting arguments

Self-Regulation
- Self-examination
- Self-correction

From Facione, P: Critical thinking: A statement of expert consensus for purpose of educational assessment and instruction. In ERIC: Research Findings and Recommendations. ERIC Document Reproduction Service, No. ED 315 423, 1992.

persistent in seeking results which are as precise as the subject and the circumstances of inquiry permit.[1]

DISPOSITIONS OF THE MODEL CRITICAL THINKER

Facione[1] outlines seven characteristics (*dispositions*) that describe the critical thinker. The critical thinker is truth seeking, open-minded, analytic, systematic, self-confident, inquisitive, and mature (Table 2–2). With these descriptives in mind, one

Table 2–2 DISPOSITIONS OF THE CRITICAL THINKER

1.	Truth seeking	Having a courageous desire for the best knowledge, even if such knowledge fails to support or undermines one's preconceptions, beliefs, or self-interests
2.	Open-minded	Tolerant of divergent views; self-monitoring for possible bias
3.	Analytic	Demanding reason and evidence; alert to problematic situations; inclined to anticipate consequences
4.	Systematic	Valuing organization, focus, and diligence to approach problems of all levels of complexity
5.	Self-confident	Trusting of one's own reasoning skills and seeing oneself as a good thinker
6.	Inquisitive	Curious and eager to acquire knowledge and learn explanations even when the applications of the knowledge are not immediately apparent
7.	Mature	Prudent in making, suspending, or revising judgment: • Aware that multiple solutions may be acceptable • Appreciates the need to reach closure even in the absence of complete knowledge

From Facione, NC and Facione, P: Workshop notes from the AAHE Assessment Forum, Washington, DC. Critical Thinking Dispositions from the California Critical Thinking Dispositions Inventory, 1992.

can pin down the basic concept of CT by incorporating basic definitions, identification of skills, and recognition of dispositions. For a comprehensive illustration, see Figure 2–1.

⇨ **Thought Prompts**

1. Practice CT by explaining the CT skills defined in the previous section.
2. Consider your own CT skill and identify ways to improve it.

APPLICATIONS OF CRITICAL THINKING TO RESPIRATORY CARE

Developing solid CT skills is essential for the RCP. Every aspect of the profession demands safe, prudent, and responsible performance from each practitioner. In the course of a single working hour, one RCP may be called on to *interpret* a complex protocol, *analyze* collected assessment data, *evaluate* the effect of a particular therapeutic regimen, *infer* that the therapeutic plan be modified, *explain* results, and make *self-corrections* all along the way. Considering this reality presents undeniable evidence in favor of promoting continuous improvement in CT skills.

The basic skills measured by the NBRC Clinical Simulation Examination (CSE) are *information gathering and decision making*. These skills are required by the RCP on a daily basis and are thus measured commercially by the NBRC. These skills are themselves a basic clustering of the skills and subskills of CT. Key indicators of CT skills required in the RC profession are found in the *content areas* of the NBRC's written examinations for entry-level *and* advanced practitioners (Table 2–3).

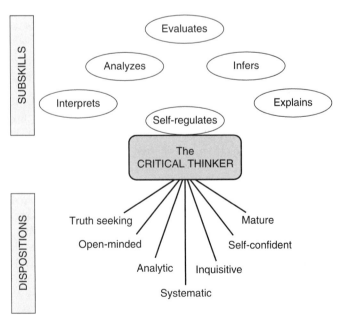

Figure 2–1. Concept map of the critical thinker. (Adapted from Facione, NC and Facione, PA: Workshop notes from the AAHE Assessment Forum, Washington, DC. Critical Thinking Dispositions from the California Critical Thinking Dispositions Inventory, 1994.)

Table 2–3 CONTENT AREAS OF THE WRITTEN CREDENTIALING EXAMINATIONS IN RESPIRATORY CARE THAT REQUIRE THINKING SKILL

Content Area

Entry Level (Certification)

I. Clinical data	• Review records; recommend diagnostic procedures. • Collect and evaluate clinical information. • Perform procedures and interpret results. • Assess therapeutic plan.
II. Equipment	• Select, obtain, and ensure cleanliness. • Assemble, check, and correct malfunctions.
III. Therapeutic procedures	• Educate patients, maintain records and communication, and control infection. • Maintain airway; mobilize and remove secretions. • Ensure ventilation. • Ensure oxygenation. • Assess patient response. • Modify therapy and make recommendations based on patient's response. • Perform emergency resuscitation.

Advanced Level (Written Registry)

I. Clinical data	• Review records; recommend diagnostic procedures. • Collect and evaluate additional clinical information. • Perform diagnostic procedures, interpret results, and assist in care plan.
II. Equipment	• Select, obtain, and ensure cleanliness. • Assemble, check for proper function, identify and/or correct malfunctions, and perform quality control.
III. Therapeutic procedures	• Evaluate, monitor, and record patient's response. • Maintain airway; remove secretions and ensure ventilation and tissue oxygenation. • Modify therapy and make recommendations based on patient's response. • Perform emergency procedures. • Assist physician, and conduct pulmonary rehabilitation and home care

Adapted from NBRC: Horizons, July/August, 1993.

⇨ Thought Prompts

3. Consider the situation of receiving an order to initiate arterial blood gas sampling and analysis on a patient. Describe the CT skills required to perform this task.

4. Make an assumption as to how the patient may respond to the blood gas procedure. Document both a positive and a negative response, and explain how the RCP should respond to each. Notice the CT skill required in each instance.

5. Choose two of the content areas from Table 2–3 and describe the CT skills required in each instance.

PRACTICING AND IMPROVING CRITICAL THINKING SKILL

Students of RC, as well as seasoned practitioners, have numerous avenues to enhance their CT skills. A good starting place is to differentiate CT from other types of thinking. Examine Table 2–4 for a comparison of *ordinary thinking* with *critical thinking*.

When we compare ordinary thinking with CT, we are in fact practicing CT. Examining the types of CT as opposed to their ordinary thinking partners promotes an understanding of the nature of CT. Other practice strategies focus on the use of the CT skills and subskills as well as on the development of the CT dispositions. A willingness to identify and adopt the CT dispositions is an excellent strategy for enhancing CT. Practice opportunities abound in *problem-based learning (PBL)* environments, where learners are free to experiment with CT techniques while enjoying access to the guidance of tutors and teachers. Other methods of learning that foster CT are listed in Table 2–5.

It should be clear that CT is not fostered by rigid reliance on one specific method but rather on a rich assortment of practice opportunities. Multiple strategies should be available for the learner to enhance CT skill. Although the list of practice strategies in Table 2–5 is lengthy, most of the methods are simple to initiate and easy to combine. PBL is the general focus of this book, but the author advocates using diverse teaching methods to sustain interest and accommodate various learning needs.

To see how the use of various strategies in combination can clarify CT instruction, let us examine the method of *structured controversy* as it might be used within a PBL environment. This technique of presenting topics for argument is easily integrated into a PBL environment. The learner is presented with data to argue from one viewpoint, given a set of guidelines, and allowed to reason and present his or her argument. Figure 2–2 is a flow diagram of the process of structured controversy.

Table 2–4 **ORDINARY THINKING VERSUS CRITICAL THINKING**

Ordinary Thinking	Critical Thinking
Guessing	Estimating
Preferring	Evaluating
Grouping	Classifying
Believing	Assuming
Inferring	Inferring logically
Associating concepts	Grasping principles
Noting relationships	Noting relationships among other relationships
Supposing	
Offering opinions without reasons	Hypothesizing
	Offering opinions with reasons
Making judgments without criteria	
	Making judgments based on criteria

Table 2–5 PRACTICE STRATEGIES FOR CRITICAL THINKING

○	Problem-based learning	The use of ill-defined problems to motivate self-investigation and regulation of the problem-solving process with expert guidance
○	Structured controversy	The use of constructed arguments for investigation
○	Management by objectives	The process of goal setting, planning, and evaluating to solve a problem
○	Self-analysis	The examination of one's performance (overall)
○	Procedure demonstration	The act of modeling a skill or behavior and explaining its components
X	Literature review	The reading and critiquing of selected pieces of literature
X	Research reporting	The inquiry into and description of a complex issue
X	Multiple-perspective viewing	The examination of various perspectives on an issue
X	Collaborative elaboration	The discussion of topics within groups or teams
X	Benchmarking	The investigation of existing models or hallmarks
X	Brainstorming	The group investigation of problems
X	Problem solving or puzzle building	The process of applying investigative procedures to solving a problem or puzzle
X	Case study analysis	The investigation of an event described in narrative form
X	Role-playing	The assuming of a function or character for purposes of understanding the role
X	Diagramming	The graphic illustration of a concept
X	Critiquing topic	The evaluation of and elaboration on a
X	Debate	The argument about a topic (less-flexible positioning than found in structured controversy)

○ = Strategies are more likely to involve all CT skills and more complex processing.
X = Strategies are less likely to involve self-regulation as a CT skill.

Participants in structured controversy should[3]:

1. Be cooperative in attitude.
2. Value the experience as a challenge.
3. Continually compare and contrast information.
4. Value and respect all those involved.

5. Maintain a supportive environment.
6. Listen critically, paraphrase, and analyze.
7. Allow for changes in perspective and avoid rigidity.
8. Practice these necessary elements:
   - Rehearsing
   - Stating own position
   - Persuading
   - Educating peers
   - Analyzing all data
   - Evaluating continually

ASSESSING CRITICAL THINKING IN RESPIRATORY CARE

As mentioned earlier, the NBRC Clinical Simulation Examination is a commercially available tool for assessing CT within the RC profession. This test divides its assessment into two main areas of CT: *information gathering* and *decision making*. The CT skills associated with information gathering include inference and self-regulation; those associated with decision making include analysis, interpretation, evaluation, and self-regulation. Often the skill of explanation is also used in each situation. A range of performance can be exhibited on this test. One can gather all of the needed information in an appropriate way (this is good), or one can gather only part of the information needed or gather it in inappropriate ways (this is not so good).

It is also possible to make correct, incorrect, or even harmful decisions on the test. The scoring ranges from a possible +3 (correct, essential) to a possible −3 (incorrect, harmful). Because CT is a flexible, varied, and progressive process, it cannot be assessed in a static way. Therefore, the key to successful completion of the test is continued practice of CT skills combined with fundamental knowledge of the discipline.

Another device to assess CT is the computer simulation, which also serves as a good practice tool. Software products often assess CT using formats that are the same as, or similar to, the Clinical Simulation Examination itself. Often a case is presented (the scenario), and then information must be gath-

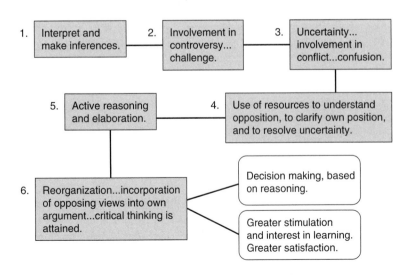

Figure 2–2. The process of structured controversy. (From Johnson, D and Johnson, R: Critical thinking through structured controversy. Educational Leadership, May, 1988, p. 62. Copyright © 1985 by ASCD. Reprinted by permission. All rights reserved.)

ered and decisions made. Scoring is often based on a scale similar to the CSE rating scale, and the examinee is often given some idea of his or her strengths and weaknesses.

Other assessments of CT and a short description of each are listed in Table 2–6. Notice that flexibility would again determine that a variety of assessments be used. Also, be aware that this list is not complete. Critical thinkers in the business of assessment are devising new methods continuously.

⇨ **Thought Prompts**

6. Do some CT practice strategies appeal to you more than others?
7. What is it about these strategies that you find particularly appealing?
8. Construct an argument that would convince someone with an opposing view that this CT strategy is a great method.

PITFALLS AND ROADBLOCKS TO CRITICAL THINKING SKILLS ENHANCEMENT

Several factors may hamper the development of CT. In general, it is some form of rigidity that interferes with good CT. This lack of flexibility may occur as a belief, a fear, or a behavior. For instance, some people believe that others are always correct in their assumptions, while the truth is that anyone can make errors. There are also those who become anxious (fearful) and find themselves unable to think clearly. And then there are those who are constantly in a rush (behavior) to "get it done," even if "it" should take a longer time for optimal results.

Table 2–7   **PITFALLS AND ROADBLOCKS TO CRITICAL THINKING**

Beliefs	Attitudes and Feelings	Behaviors
Overestimations	Anxiety or fear	Hastiness
Incorrect generalizations	Fatigue	Disorganization
Emotional tie-ins	Expectancies	Avoidance
False beliefs	Rigidity	Entrapment
Doubt	Immaturity	Aggression
Incorrect assumptions	Lack of motivation	Passivity
Conformity	Anger	Subordination
Subjectivity	Insecurity	Dominance

The other major stumbling block to development of CT is a lack of information. Without possessing the basic knowledge of a discipline, one cannot hope to develop high-level, well-organized thoughts about the subject. The acquisition of discipline-specific knowledge is a developmental process, in which more basic facts are understood first and more complex concepts are acquired over time. To view a more complete collection of *pitfalls and roadblocks* that interfere with CT, read and consider Table 2–7.

All critical thinkers are likely to stumble into one of these pitfalls on occasion. Often simply being aware of potential problems can help people avoid them. Maintaining a firm focus on the use of evidence, performing continuous self-correction (improvement), and having a sensitivity to the context of an issue enhance the use of CT.

⇨ **Thought Prompts**

9. Choose one item from each category in Table 2–7 and describe an RC situation in which this problem could occur.
10. How might you adapt to such a situation?

EXPERTS VERSUS NOVICES

There are many differences between the way experts approach and solve problems and the way novices do. The main contrast is in the application of CT to the situation. Experts have more experience and, therefore, a larger knowledge base. Experts also have had more practice at CT within their domain. Novices, on the other hand, are generally more dependent on guidelines and rules and are less likely to be willing to trust that their CT ability will "handle" the situation.[4] In the RC profession, the novice will approach and attain expert status when his or her CT skills develop to the point that they are recognized as dependable. Figure 2–3 is a comparison chart of the expert versus novice characteristics.

The combination of characteristics attributed to the expert contributes to what is known as "intuition." *Intuition* allows the expert to make solid hunches based on cues received, which is essential to expert decision making. In the same situation the novice relies on a base of information for decision

Table 2–6   **ASSESSMENTS OF CRITICAL THINKING**

Clinical simulations	NBRC commercial test
Computer simulations	Software presenting an RC case and evaluating information gathering and decision making
Portfolio examination	Assessment of a collection of works, thoughts, and/or creations
Outcome measures	Assessment of the end result of a project
Goal and objective examination	Assessment of the goals and objectives set and measured by the learner
Peer evaluation	Peers and assessing other members of a group, using criteria
Scoring of argument	Rating of the power of an argument as to reasoning, communication, and outcome
Communication	Scoring and critiquing of written or spoken communication as to CT criteria
Multiple-choice testing	Assessment using the traditional multiple-answer format*
Other commercial tests	California Critical Thinking Skills Test, Ennis-Weir Critical Thinking Essay, Watson-Glaser CT Appraisal, Cornell CT Test

*One interesting twist to the multiple-choice testing theme is to analyze why the wrong answers are incorrect and to explain this analysis in oral or written form.

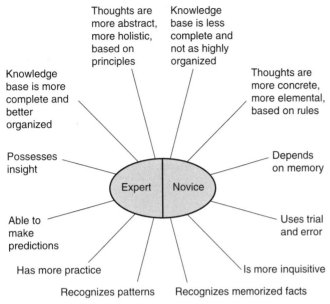

Figure 2–3. The expert versus the novice critical thinking approach.

making. As the novice gains experience, he or she evolves into the expert.

Two events in the thinking process are critical to the discussion of *expert versus novice thinking.* One event, called *incubation,* corresponds to the time in which a thought or idea is contemplated and related to other known variables. This incubation period allows for focusing on the problem at hand. During the incubation period an event called *metacognition* occurs. This term refers to the process of thinking about one's thinking. In a sense it is the basis of the self-check system in thinking. These events in CT are essential to the self-regulatory process. With continued practice, the incubation period for related problems will decrease and the CT skill will improve. The expert thought process is made up of shorter incubation periods with more efficient metacognitive activity. This accounts for the frequent occasions when an expert is asked to explain how the solution to a problem was found and he or she confesses that the solution "just came" to him or her. As with any efficient process or machine, there are times when the activity appears effortless.

Whether one views thinking patterns in terms of outcomes or elements, the basic fact remains the same: The practice and level of CT ability within the profession differentiate the expert from the novice and allow for greater working efficiency and improved quality of care.

⇨ **Thought Prompts**

11. Discuss the ways in which experts and novices differ. Use your own words, and create examples within RC to clarify your meaning.
12. How are experts and novices alike?

Summary

This chapter focuses on the process of CT, its associated skills and dispositions, and its application to RC. Key content areas in which CT skill is assessed in the NBRC credentialing system are discussed. Comparison between CT and ordinary thinking is made. Various strategies for practicing and assessing CT are highlighted. Pitfalls and roadblocks to good CT are mentioned. Finally, the differences between expert and novice thinking are examined.

References

1. Facione, P: Critical thinking: A statement of expert consensus for purpose of educational assessment and instruction. In ERIC: Research Findings and Recommendations. ERIC Document Reproduction Service, No. ED 315 423, Atlanta, 1992.
2. Facione, NC and Facione, PA: Workshop notes from the AAHE Assessment Forum, Washington, DC. Critical Thinking Dispositions from the California Critical Thinking Dispositions Inventory, 1994.
3. Johnson, D and Johnson, R: Critical thinking through structured controversy. Educational Leadership, May 1988, pp. 58–64.
4. Klein, S: Learning, ed 2. McGraw-Hill, New York, 1991, p. 318.

Suggested Reading

Chaffee, J: Thinking Critically, ed 3. Houghton Mifflin, Boston, 1991.

Halpern, D: Thought and Knowledge: An Introduction to Critical Thinking. L. Erlbaum Associates, 1989.

Meyer, D: The use of literature in training respiratory care practitioners. The AARC Distinguished Papers Monograph 2:45–52, 1993.

Mishoe, S: Critical thinking, education preparation and development of respiratory care practitioners. The AARC Distinguished Papers Monograph 2:29–43, 1993.

Ormrod, J: Human Learning. Merrill, New York, 1991.

Paul, R: Critical Thinking, ed. 3. The Foundation for Critical Thinking, Cotati, CA, 1990.

PRACTICE QUESTIONS

In answering the following, explain why the incorrect answers are incorrect.

1. CT may be enhanced by:
   A. Practicing goal setting
   B. Learning basic information about a discipline
   C. Reading and commenting on literature
   D. Examining one's own performance
   E. All of the above

2. Critical thinkers perform all of the following skills as an example of their ability except:
   A. Identifying arguments
   B. Recalling complete data charts
   C. Justifying procedures
   D. Self-correcting
   E. Clarifying meaning

3. When faced with a clinical decision of considerable importance, an RCP who is skilled in CT would:

A. Make the correct choice as a result of good CT.
B. Approach the decision in a systematic way.
C. Seek the truth through data collection.
D. Make many inquiries.
E. Do all of the above.

4. Which of the following is descriptive of CT?
   I. Estimating
   II. Preferring
   III. Believing
   IV. Assuming
   V. Grasping principles
      A. I, II, and III
      B. I, III, and V
      C. I, III, IV, and V
      D. I, IV, and V
      E. I, II, III, IV, and V

5. Of the following, which are criteria for assessing competence in CT?
   A. Competence in using the CT subskills
   B. Benchmarking
   C. Problem-based learning
   D. Brainstorming
   E. All of the above

6. The incubation period that occurs when a problem is given without its answer promotes:
   A. Controversy
   B. The assessment of CT
   C. Metacognition
   D. Decay of motivation
   E. All of the above

7. To maintain a structured controversy, participants should do all of the following except:
   A. Be prepared to gain consensus.
   B. Value the experience as a challenge.
   C. Listen critically.
   D. Rehearse.
   E. Be cooperative in attitude.

8. Those who achieve expert status are least likely to:
   A. Identify patterns and relationships.
   B. Pay strict attention to memorized facts.
   C. Think in abstract terms.
   D. Have insight into problems within the discipline.
   E. View problems in a holistic manner.

9. Of the following, who would have the least inhibition to CT?
   A. A person who is very excited about an event
   B. Someone who has just had an aggressive argument
   C. Someone who is having a busy workday
   D. Someone who has ingrained beliefs about the topic
   E. Someone who commits wholeheartedly to his or her idea on the subject

ACTIVITIES

1. Perform a self-evaluation. Use the following evaluation as an organizer:

Criteria	RATINGS					
	(lower)	1	2	3	4	5 (higher)
Skill:						
analysis						
interpretation						
evaluation						
inference						
explanation						
self-regulation						

2. Find resources that allow you to practice your CT skills and evaluate their usefulness. (Try rating them according to interest, enjoyment, and effectiveness. Add criteria that you find pertinent.)

3. Initiate a discussion about CT, and try to gain a consensus concerning its importance in the practice of RC. (Perhaps a group meeting or class would serve this purpose.)

3 | Assessment in Respiratory Care: A Cognitive Approach

Learning Objectives

After reading the chapter and performing the activities within it, the learner will be able to:

- Identify assessment as a process.
- Integrate the concept of critical thinking (CT) into the assessment process.
- Describe a systematic approach for physical assessment.
- Recognize the attributes of skillful assessment practices.
- Identify basic assessment skills.
- Identify complex assessment techniques.
- Identify the factors that regulate the assessment process.
- Apply the use of assessment findings to therapeutic intervention, care planning, and continuous quality improvement.
- Identify special populations as pertaining to assessment in RC.
- Elaborate on the linkage existing between assessment and outcome evaluation.

Key Words and Phrases

Assessing by exception
Assessment
Assessment and outcome
  evaluations
Basic versus complex
  assessments
Checklist approach
Chronological review
Communicative
Comprehensive
Critical thinking (CT)
Cumulative
Data analysis

Ethical and standard
  practices
Evaluation
Head-to-toe
  examination
Historical events
Information gathering
Modifying plans
Norm based
Objective documentation
Opportunistic
Quality assurance and
  improvement

Regulation of the
  assessment process
Resource based
Special populations
Systematic
Systematic pulmonary
  assessment
Systems approach
Therapeutic interventions
Therapeutic plan
Treatment assessments

WHAT IS ASSESSMENT?

Assessment in RC is the collecting of information about a given situation. Assessments help to form the professional evaluations that develop from that collected information. For instance, one may *assess* that a patient's breath sounds are absent over the right upper lobe. Other assessments, such as noting dyspnea, tachycardia, and a decrease in dynamic compliance, may be added to the original breath sound finding. This information may then be combined with the knowledge that the patient had a central venous catheter placed 5 minutes ear-

lier. After the assessments are collected and analyzed, the *evaluation* (or *judgment*) may be made that a pneumothorax is present.

Assessment involves *critical thinking* (CT) on the part of the RCP. The use of CT allows assessments to be grouped into meaningful relationships, giving direction to further investigation or action. The assessment process, using CT as a core, is composed of making observations, selecting information, recognizing patterns and relationships in the data, and then analyzing all the components as a whole. The analysis yields evaluative decisions regarding the *therapeutic plan* of patient care. In essence it is through this process that RCPs *decide* which data will be considered, as well as how the data will be used. As illustrated in Figure 3–1, assessment is actually a skill born of CT.[1]

By applying CT skills to the assessment process, the RCP continuously uses the information presented in each case in a cumulative manner, continuously collecting and using feedback from each situation. Attention is paid to any clues that may have meaning to the case. Often, although not always, these clues group into clusters that are representative of a pathological condition.[2] The assessments mentioned earlier that support the diagnostic evaluation of pneumothorax are an example of a cluster of clues. Rarely does a practitioner make a patient evaluation based on only one assessment. Such decisions are generally the result of many bits of collected information, which are analyzed and then interpreted.

Thorough assessment of the patient involves *information gathering* and *data analysis*. Evaluations are then based on this assessment process. This thoughtful approach to assessment ensures that patient care is delivered in a safe and reasonable fashion. Consider the following scenario as an example of practicing assessment as a function of CT:

SCENARIO

A practitioner enters the patient's room in response to a newly received order for consultation on a postoperative patient. The RCP immediately takes note of the overall picture, including direct observation of the patient and the surroundings. The RCP notes that the patient appears drowsy and somewhat uncomfortable but concludes that this is an expected finding. As the visual overview continues, the practitioner recalls seeing documentation of an axillary temperature of 100.5°F in the medical chart and notices that the heart rate registering on the bedside pulse oximeter is reading 130 bpm with a saturation of 94 percent. Before even beginning auscultation or seeing a chest x-ray, the practitioner is inferring that atelectasis may be present in this patient. The practitioner has put together a "cluster" of evidence pointing to atelectasis. The cluster consists of postoperative condition, elevated temperature, accelerated heart rate, and decreased saturation.

The practitioner now proceeds with a physical assessment and checks to see if other signs, such as weak cough, basilar crackles, limited or unilateral chest expansion, dull percussion note, or decreased vital capacity, are present.[3] Note that assumptions are made based on reasonable evidence, but other significant findings may alter the assumptions. The process of planning therapy for the patient in this case will be linked to the assessments, assumptions, and decisions made during this initial visit.

Skillful assessment of the respiratory patient is *systematic*, *comprehensive*, and *cumulative* in nature. An *opportunistic* approach should be employed. It involves open and clear *com-*

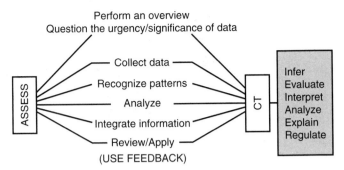

Figure 3–1. Concept map of assessment as a function of critical thinking (CT). Note the interrelationship between the CT skills and the process of assessment.

munication among the practitioner, the patient, the physician, the nurse, and other professionals involved. Careful attention must be paid to the *historical events* of the case, as well as to the current information being gathered. The RCP must be mindful of the *ethical and standard practices* of assessment and understand the *norms* associated with these practices. He or she should also consider the use of *multiple resources* for gathering patient data. A clear understanding of the norms applying to the situation should also be incorporated into the assessment process. *Objective documentation* and storage of information also must be considered to properly maintain the patient record. Skillful assessment practices are:

- Systematic
- Comprehensive
- Cumulative
- Opportunistic
- Based on communication
- Based on history
- Based on ethical and standard practices for assessing client status
- *Resource based*
- Based on an understanding of norms associated with assessments
- Recorded in objective documentation

See also Figure 3–2.

A Systematic Approach

It is most probable that RCPs use nearly all of the assessment techniques that modern medicine has to offer. Therefore, the differences in approaching assessment are vast. However, one consistent element remains within all good assessment approaches—systematicity. To use a *systematic* approach is to follow a plan that ensures collection of data in all pertinent areas. Being systematic in assessment ensures consistency and reduces the risk of overlooking significant findings. Systematic approaches include the following:

Head-to-Toe Approach (or Toe-to-Head). Conducting assessments in the order of "appearance" on the body—scanning from the head to the feet, or vice versa. For example,

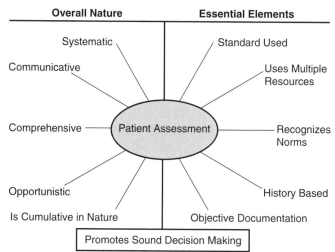

Figure 3–2. Concept map of the assessment process factors.

starting at the head, one may perform neurological evaluations, communication assessment, and oral inspection, as well as many other assessments.[4]

Systems Approach. Approaching assessment by examining the body according to its organ systems. Obviously in most RC instances, pulmonary assessment is of highest importance. However, one should not overlook significant evidence derived from assessing other organ systems, particularly cardiac, renal, and neurological.

Chronological Review. Assessments made using a timeframe. For instance, the overall assessment should begin with a look at the client's history and then proceed in a linear fashion to the present.

Assessing by Exception. Making assessments regarding unusual events, such as an unexpected patient response to treatment. This type of assessment is most notable in the case of routine patient monitoring that leads to a significant finding.

Checklist Approach. The assessment process performed according to a list. The practitioner proceeds through the assessment process by following a written guideline. Commonly, key descriptive terms are listed and the practitioner may choose the term that most closely fits the situation.

Treatment Assessments. The monitoring of a set of parameters. Often the RCP will see a patient more than once during a working shift. This usually occurs when multiple treatments are required. Rather than repeating previous assessments, the RCP monitors a specific "set" of parameters (pulse, breath sounds, etc.) that are related to the treatment being given or that are representative of the treatment outcome. (See Chap. 5 for further information on treatment outcome.)

Systematic Pulmonary Assessment. Common pulmonary assessments including the gathering of information on heart rate, respiratory rate, auscultation, skin color, level of consciousness, record review, consultation with other professionals, examination of chest x-rays, and performance of other relative examinations.[5]

Although no single method is advocated over others, some combination of methods is usually the most suitable. Borrowing from each of the approaches creates an assessment model that is comprehensive, consistent, and useful in producing desired patient outcomes. This creativity reinforces the disposition of being open-minded and flexible, allowing many tactics to be integrated into one's practice.

⇨ **Thought Prompts**

1. How does systematicity promote effective assessment skill?
2. Create a logical argument (a few sentences) defending the use of combining several of the systematic assessment approaches noted in this section.
3. Explain the application of CT to the assessment process. How does CT ensure the quality of the process?

A Comprehensive Evaluation

To collect appropriate information in a particular case, the RCP needs to take an overall "look" at the situation and all the events surrounding it. This thoroughness should be ensured with the use of a systematic approach to assessment. An example of a comprehensive assessment is the complete history and physical examination routinely performed on patients who are newly admitted to a hospital or clinic.

A Cumulative Process

Assessment is a cumulative process. Each part of each case is factored in to create the whole picture. One must always continue the assessment process in light of the information that has already been gathered about a particular situation. The additive nature of assessment creates the database within a patient case. The entire medical record of a patient represents the cumulative collection of information in a case.

An Opportunistic Approach

To allow continuous and pertinent information collection, the RCP must remain opportunistic. That is to say that significant data may present at *any time;* therefore the practitioner must be alert to changes at all times. When RCPs collect and use information as it manifests, they are being opportunistic. This allows data to be used to their full advantage as soon as they become available.

Open and Clear Communication Channels

To effectively work with clients and gather information from them, the RCP must be a most efficient communicator. Note that communication involves both sending *and* receiving messages. Emphasis should be placed on listening and speaking skills. Good communication requires attention to detail. Practice in CT skills will facilitate one's ability to attend to details and form inferences from the data.

Historical Review of the Client and Problem(s)

In assessing a current situation, the RCP should always refer back in time, either by interviewing the client, family, and others or by consulting documents covering past events. A historical perspective also contributes to projections of future events.

Use of Ethical and Standard Techniques

To maintain one's competence and integrity, the use of standard tools must be incorporated into practice. Each RCP should practice according to the accepted norms and guidelines of the profession. In patient assessment, care should be taken to ensure that the patient's rights are protected and considered at each step in the process. Confidentiality and respect are key factors in ethical practice. Knowledge of ethical principles such as autonomy, veracity, maleficence, beneficence, and justice is also essential to skillful practice. Using standard tools promotes effectiveness by maintaining quality of care, minimizing patient and practitioner risks, and enhancing organization. The standard practice tools associated with pulmonary assessment include observation, palpation, auscultation, and percussion. Current clinical practice guidelines and health care standards such as the patient's bill of rights should establish the framework for all RC practice.

Multiple Resources

Assessment is a comprehensive process and thus is not limited to a specific setting. To collect all necessary information on a case, the RCP must consult:

- The patient, family, and significant others, by interview and examination
- The medical record
- Other health practitioners (doctor, nurse)
- Diagnostic services (labs, imaging)
- References (medical dictionary, journals)

There are certainly times when this primary list must be extended, but these sources are the core of meaningful assessment.

Knowledge of Pathological Norms

Practitioners cannot interpret data if they are not knowledgeable about them. For instance, to accurately collect and analyze information about a client's breath sounds, one must distinguish between "normal" and the "unusual." To make clinical decisions and become proficient in assessing the patient, RCPs must possess knowledge about pathophysiology. They must be acquainted with common disorders affecting the pulmonary system and be mindful of the assessments associated with them.

A flexibility should also exist to allow room for exceptions. For example, clear (vesicular) breath sounds are the normal breath sound over healthy lung tissue, while wheezes are abnormal sounds. However, there are times when a certain amount of wheezing is "normal" for a particular patient (for instance, those with tracheal stenosis).[6] To make this judgment, the RCP must have a truly good grasp of the concept of "normal" assessment findings and a highly competent skill level in comprehensive assessment. The RCP also must possess the thinking skills that promote clinical insight into individual patient cases. It is precisely this truth-seeking perspective that enhances high-level assessment skills.

Objective Data Collection

For collection of information about clients to be organized in a meaningful way, there must be a system for its storage. Most commonly this system involves documents found in a medical record, either written on paper or entered into a computerized system. This system organizes information and ensures that it is processed in a consistently useful fashion. It also maintains access to records for those needing it.

Information collected in RC should be reported in an objective fashion. Objective language is impartial and explains the measure of something. For instance, instead of documenting that the patient appeared short of breath, one could record that marked use of accessory muscles, tachypnea, and upper chest retractions were noted. Mention of the patient's subjective complaint of shortness of breath is also worthy of notation. See Figure 3–2 for an overview of the assessment process.

⇨ **Thought Prompt**
4. Consider the advantages and disadvantages of using reference materials (books, journals) during the clinical practice of RC. Record your thoughts in writing.

COMMON ASSESSMENT DATA SOURCES

As stated, RCPs may access a tremendous variety of information regarding a given situation. Current literature holds a wealth of knowledge regarding the various sources of assessment data (see suggested readings). In an effort to categorize and present a "bird's-eye view" of many of the potential sources of assessments, Figure 3–3 was developed.[7–10] This overall presentation will be referred to throughout the cases

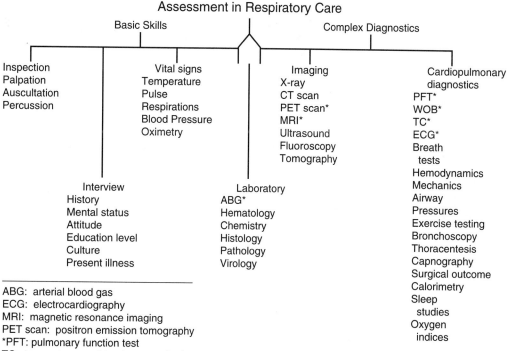

Figure 3–3. Concept map of common assessment categories in respiratory care.

presented in this book. This collection, like sound CT, is not an exclusive list but, rather, an overall picture of the common sources of assessment data.

⇨ Thought Prompts

5. Assume you are assessing a patient (for instance, listening to breath sounds or observing muscle use). In what ways does your assessment process change when unexpected (abnormal) results are found?
6. How do unusual findings affect RC planning of treatment and monitoring?
7. Create clinical examples of instances that would require recommending changes in therapy based on assessment findings involving:
   A. Patient's physical changes
   B. Negative patient changes associated with treatment
   C. Problems with malfunctioning equipment

REGULATION OF THE ASSESSMENT PROCESS

The assessment process is ongoing and continuous. The information collected through assessment must be used in constructive, meaningful ways. Assessment should have a focus and some objective goal should exist to make assessment purposeful. Assessment should be performed with the interests of the patient as a primary goal and with concern for the com-

munity or the facility the patient is in. For instance, one should collect all pertinent information about a patient while maintaining patient safety. At the same time, cost-effective use of available resources should also be considered to provide high-quality service. The description of the assessment process, noted earlier (systematic, cumulative, etc.), highlights the essential ingredients in performing quality assessments that remain cost effective. The addition of the KIS method (Keep It Simple) may complete the list of descriptives. When faced with what at times seems like endless potential for gathering information, striving to be resourceful and as noninvading as possible is critical to the RC process.

⇨ Thought Prompt
8. Make assumptions regarding the regulation of the assessment process. Use the example of a trauma victim dependent on mechanical ventilation. Consider ways to minimize assessment costs, ways to minimize risks, and ways to maximize the benefit associated with the process.

APPLICATIONS OF ASSESSMENT DATA

Therapeutic Interventions

Assessment of patients is often focused on the therapeutic regimen they are undergoing. For example, when a patient receives a nebulized medication treatment, assessments are made concerning the indication, effect, and outcome of the treatment. In such a case, data are gathered supporting (or negating) treatment indication, such as the presence of wheezing. There is also investigation into the treatment effect, such as a monitoring of vital signs. Then treatment outcome is assessed to lend evidence supporting positive, negative, or neutral end result. In our nebulized medication case, we might find that our patient's wheezing clears and that obvious accessory muscle use ceases. In more complex forms of therapy, more complex assessments must be made. As seen in Figure 3–3, there are numerous tools for use in assessing patients. These tools must be used appropriately to provide information that must then be interpreted, analyzed, and used in further planning.

Therapeutic Planning and Recommendations

Once data are collected, they undergo interpretation by the RCP and then serve as the basis for creating the RC plan (see Chap. 5). Once this plan is developed, the analysis of collected information may result in three distinct planning outcomes, as follows:

1. Evidence may support maintaining the present plan and its associated treatments and monitors.
2. Evidence may support either changing the plan by recommending suitable alternatives or *modifying the present plan* by adding or deleting certain treatments or monitors.
3. Evidence may support discontinuing the present plan because of its lack of patient benefit. (For instance, a patient progresses and no longer requires the service, treatment, or monitor.)

In making assessments pertaining to care planning, reasoning must be heavily employed. This CT strategy may follow a relatively simple pattern. In assessing the RC plan, the practitioner might use a framework such as that presented in Table 3–1. Always bear in mind that sound CT facilitates sound practice.

Patient Equipment and Its Service Quality

When considering the assessment of equipment use and function, one can never overestimate the importance of following the manufacturer's recommendations for use and maintenance of the equipment.[11] To "check" equipment function, the manufacturer supplies guidelines that are systematic, comprehensive, and specific to the equipment itself. All policies and procedures concerning each piece of equipment should be maintained and updated accordingly. Of course, all service and maintenance should be documented, and equipment performance should be monitored on an ongoing basis. Equip-

---

Table 3–1 EXAMPLES OF ASSESS AND EVALUATE STRATEGIES

Assessing

Ask probing questions: "Is this treatment benefiting the patient?"

Make confirming statements: "Wheezing disappeared after treatment."

or

"Wheezing continues after treatment."

Evaluating

Regulate the plan: "This regimen is working to dilate the airway; we should continue with our strategy."

or

"The patient is progressing well. I recommend discontinuing nebulized medication and beginning the metered dose inhaler protocol."

or

"The treatment is not having the intended effect on the patient. I recommend a change in medication."

---

ment reliability may be ensured by using performance checks before and after use. All malfunctioning or suspect equipment should be labeled accordingly and placed in a specified area for further inspection, repair, or replacement.

When assessing equipment for proper function, use a systematic approach, continuously analyzing the form and function of the equipment. Always ensure patient safety by assessing the patient before, during (at specific intervals, if equipment use is continuous), and after equipment use. One way to prevent mishaps when you suspect an equipment malfunction is to separate the "danger" from the patient. Whether the equipment is as simple as a metered dose inhaler or as complex as a microprocessor ventilator, whenever possible, remove the suspect equipment from the immediate patient environment. When the immediate risk is minimized, a thorough assessment of the equipment may be made without risk to patient safety. This may often mean that suitable equipment must be substituted either temporarily or permanently.

Continuous Quality Improvement

Assessment is the core of evaluating and promoting *continuous quality improvement* (CQI) in RC. As part of the CQI process, the RCP assesses patients, equipment, and services, leading to evaluations. The assessment process is ongoing, objective, cumulative, and goal oriented. When data are collected in a focused manner and meaningful decisions are made, the quality of care may be enhanced on a continuous basis, rather than on an "end-of-the-line" basis. In other words, it is better to prevent problems than to solve them.

ASSESSMENT OF SPECIAL POPULATIONS

The Neonatal Population

Neonates, be assured, are not small adults. They have distinct characteristics that predispose them to many risks that do not threaten adults. One such risk concerns thermoregulation. When assessing the neonate in any situation, the RCP must pay careful attention to maintaining the neonate's body warmth (called *maintenance of neutral thermal environment*).[12] This problem is associated with the infant's body surface-to-weight ratio, as well as several developmental factors. Thermoregulation is only one example of uniqueness in this population. Further examples are featured in Chapters 17 and 18. For further reference on specific assessment findings in this population, refer to the suggested readings at the end of this chapter.

The Pediatric Population

Again, this population represents a significant collection of assessment data that differs from that of adults. Most assessment differences between adult and pediatric patients stem from differences in body weight and body surface area. However, psychoemotional differences also exist, and they should dictate the assessment approach to the pediatric patient as well. Children require care suited to their needs. One cannot overlook the importance of focusing assessment and care on the individual child. Maturity level and emotional need must be considered as the pediatric patient is examined.[13] To maintain communication and promote understanding, one must use age-appropriate language. For specific references on this population, refer to the suggested readings at the end of this chapter.

The Geriatric Population

Geriatric patients may have visual and hearing impairments that require attention to promote meaningful assessment. For instance, large-print written documents may be helpful for visually impaired patients, and speaking carefully may be helpful for verbal communication with hearing impaired patients.[14] As in other special populations, age-associated norms must be examined and incorporated into the assessments. As with all patient populations, individual attention is critical to proper assessment. Again, refer to the suggested readings for more detailed information on the geriatric population.

The Home Care Population

In the ever-growing home care sector of RC, assessment of the patient, family, and the environment is crucial. The home RCP has a great responsibility to assess the patient thoroughly. The degree of monitoring in the home is far less than that in a hospital. Thus, greater responsibility rests with the home care providers.

Home care assessment areas that require special emphasis are environmental safety, activities of daily living, and psychosocial issues.[15] Assessment of the total patient and environment is crucial to safe and successful RC of the patient in the home (see suggested readings).

Multicultural Environments

To practice RC in today's health care arena, one must be sensitive to cultural diversity. People from various cultures hold a multitude of beliefs. Communication and emotion may be conveyed in unfamiliar contexts through spoken words or subtle gestures. Each RCP should be mindful of the wealth of multicultural diversity, especially within his or her own community, and strive to maintain an open perspective and sensitive demeanor.

⇨ **Thought Prompts**

9. Consider how knowledge of standard assessments plays an essential part in dealing with members of the neonatal, pediatric, and geriatric populations. What standards may require adjustment in considering these populations?
10. Identify a variety of cultural beliefs focused on the medical delivery system. Discuss ways to enhance the multicultural aspects of your own practice.

ASSESSMENT AND OUTCOME EVALUATION

In attempting to measure the outcome of a particular case, the RCP must summon a variety of skills. No skill is more central to evaluating patient outcome from therapeutic interventions than that of gathering assessment data. Whether we monitor breath sounds or compute the work of our patients' breathing, the collected information will serve as the measure of success or failure in a given instance. When assessing patients, the RCP must maintain a keen focus on those cues that represent the outcome of therapy. With such cues in mind, assessment can be maintained as an effective tool in the outcome management of patient care (see Chap. 4).

⇨ **Thought Prompts**

11. Describe the relationship between patient assessment and outcome management.
12. How can high-level assessment skill promote better patient outcomes?

Summary

This chapter focuses on the assessment process. The integration of sound CT serves as the cornerstone of good assessment skill. Several assessment systems are considered, along with an integrated approach. Common assessment categories are listed for review. Regulation and application of assessments are explained, and special populations are noted. Last, the linkage between assessment and outcome evaluation is described.

References

1. Carnevali, D and Thomas, M: Diagnostic Reasoning and Treatment Decision Making in Nursing. JB Lippincott, Philadelphia, 1993, p. 124.
2. Scheffer, BK: Critical Thinking in Nursing, An Interactive Approach. JB Lippincott, Philadelphia, 1995, p. 121.
3. Farzan, S: A Concise Handbook of Respiratory Disease, ed 3. Appleton & Lange, Stamford, CT, 1992, p. 243.
4. Fuller, J and Schaller-Ayers, J: Health Assessment: A Nursing Approach. JB Lippincott, Philadelphia, 1994, p. 31.
5. AARC: Respiratory Care Uniform Reporting Manual, ed 3. Dallas, 1989, p. 9.
6. Khadra, I and Braun, S: Upper airway obstruction. In: Braun, S: Pulmonary Medicine. Elsevier, New York, 1989, p. 141.
7. Smith, JP and Pierson, DJ: Diagnostic imaging. In: Kacmarek, R: Foundations of Respiratory Care. Churchill Livingstone Inc, New York, 1992, p. 593.
8. Chu, LW and Wilkins, RL: Clinical laboratory studies. In: Wilkins, RL, Sheldon, RL and Krider, SJ: Clinical Assessment in Respiratory Care. Mosby, St. Louis, 1990, p. 56.
9. Pleval, DJ and Didier, EP: A guide to patient assessment for respiratory care practitioners. In: Barnes, TA: Core Textbook of Respiratory Care Practice. Mosby, St. Louis, 1994, p. 91.
10. Wilkins, RL: Techniques of physical examination. In: Wilkins, RL, Sheldon, RL and Krider, SJ: Clinical Assessment in Respiratory Care. Mosby, St. Louis, 1990, p. 26.
11. Russel, G: Risky business. Advance for Managers of Respiratory Care 3:29, 1994.
12. Aloan, CA: Respiratory Care of the Newborn. JB Lippincott, Philadelphia, 1987, p. 97.
13. Whaley, LF and Wong, DL: Communication and health assessment of the child and family. In: Nursing Care of Infants and Children, ed 4. Mosby, St. Louis, 1991, p. 1379.
14. Giordano, J: Assessing the need of geriatric patients at home. AARC Times, November, 1993, p. 52.
15. Giordano, S: Current and future role of respiratory care practitioners in home care. Respiratory Care 39:321, 1994.

Suggested Reading

Aloan, CA: Respiratory Care of the Newborn: A Clinical Manual. JB Lippincott, Philadelphia, 1987.

Barnhart, S and Czervinske, MP: Perinatal and Pediatric Respiratory Care. WB Saunders, Philadelphia, 1995.

Carrol, C: Legal Issues and Ethical Dilemmas in Respiratory Care. FA Davis, Philadelphia, 1996.

Farzan, S: A Concise Handbook of Respiratory Disease, ed 3. Appleton & Lange, Stamford, CT, 1992.

Kacmarek, R: Foundations of Respiratory Care. Churchill Livingstone Inc, New York, 1992.

Koff, PB, Eitzman, DV and Neu, J: Neonatal and Pediatric Respiratory Care. Mosby, St. Louis, 1988.

Lucas, J, Golish J, Sleeper G et al: Home Respiratory Care. Appleton & Lange, Norwalk CT, 1988.

May, D: Rehabilitation and Continuity of Care in Pulmonary Disease. Mosby. St. Louis, 1991.

Olds, S, London, M and Ladewig, P: Maternal Newborn Nursing, ed 4. Addison-Wesley, Redwood, CA, 1992.

Scanlan, C, Spearman, C and Sheldon, R: Egan's Fundamentals of Respiratory Care, ed 6. Mosby, St. Louis, 1995.

Whitaker K: Comprehensive Perinatal and Pediatric Respiratory Care. Delmar, Albany, NY, 1992.

Wilkins, RL and Dexter, JR: Respiratory Disease: A Case Study Approach to Patient Care, ed 2. FA Davis, Philadelphia, 1997.

PRACTICE QUESTIONS

1. All of the following are components of the assessment process except:
   A. Skillful communication
   B. Cumulative addition of information
   C. Recognition of pertinent historical data
   D. Detection of unusual events
   E. Formation of judgments

2. Which of the following would you use to perform a limited pulmonary assessment of a patient receiving a positive expiratory pressure treatment?
   I. ABG
   II. Respiratory rate and pattern
   III. Level of consciousness
   IV. Capnography
   V. Auscultation
   A. I, II, III, IV, and V
   B. II, III, IV, and V
   C. II, III, and IV
   D. II, III, and V
   E. I, III, and V

3. Which of the following are good sources of data regarding the patient's medical history?
   A. The medical record
   B. The patient interview
   C. A consultation with the primary care physician
   D. A and B
   E. A, B, and C

4. Which of the following is most likely to produce evidence of the outcome of therapy?
   A. The physician discontinues the treatment.
   B. The patient states he or she is feeling better.
   C. Therapy is documented on a continuous basis.
   D. The therapeutic objective is met.
   E. Complete assessment is performed.

5. Which of the following is an example of an assessment norm?
   A. A tuberculosis patient coughs productively.
   B. An infant exhibits central cyanosis.
   C. A COPD patient states he or she has chest pain.
   D. A postop patient complains of left-sided numbness.
   E. A pneumonia patient produces copious amounts of bloody sputum.

6. All of the following are objectives of clinical assessment except:
   A. Maintain patient's safety.
   B. Collect pertinent information.
   C. Maximize efficient use of resources.
   D. Minimize patient and practitioner risks.
   E. Maximize use of invasive diagnostic tools.

7. Which of the following is the appropriate sequence in the assessment process?
   I. Identifying the problem and possible causes
   II. Reassessing the current plan
   III. Making inferences as to the problem at hand
   IV. Creating plans for dealing with the problem
   V. Collecting data central to the problem
      A. V, IV, III, and I
      B. I, III, V, and II
      C. II, V, I, IV, and III
      D. IV, V, III, II, and I
      E. I, II, IV, III, and V

8. The core ingredient of RC assessment is:
   A. Diagnostic testing
   B. Observation
   C. CT
   D. Standard comparisons
   E. Continuous quality improvement

9. All RC assessment should be:
   A. Therapy oriented
   B. Process oriented, thorough, and complete
   C. Ongoing, continuous, and objectively oriented
   D. Communication based and diagnostic
   E. Oriented toward making recommendations

4 | Evaluation in Respiratory Care

Learning Objectives

After reading the chapter and performing the activities within it, the learner will be able to:

- Identify and define the process of evaluation in RC.
- Recognize the need for ongoing evaluation processes.
- Identify four target areas for evaluation in RC.
- Recognize two general perspectives of evaluation used in health care.
- Recognize the link between evaluation and quality improvement.
- Describe outcome management, and relate it to the evaluation process in RC.

Key Words and Phrases

Competency evaluation
Compliance with standards
Cost effectiveness
CQI
Customer satisfaction
Evaluation targets
Focused inquiry
Indicators
Outcome management
Patient condition
Patient or client survey

Peer review
Performance appraisal
Process and outcome
  evaluations
Reliability
Risk analysis
Self-evaluation
Therapeutic response
  and regimen
Time utilization
Validity

WHAT IS THE EVALUATION PROCESS?

Evaluation, an ongoing process in which assessments form the basis of judgments,[1] is a fundamental unit of the RC department's structure. Without a continuous, overall, and well-maintained evaluation system, the avenues for improving the quality of service and the working environment would be quite narrow. Evaluation is the tool with which RCPs investigate, form conclusions, and then make recommendations about their professional endeavors. Few areas of the profession are exempt from needing evaluation and subsequent improvement.

The basic steps in the evaluation process are planning the evaluation, collecting the data, analyzing the data, reporting and/or documenting the information, and applying the results to improve or maintain quality.

To be more specific, evaluation is *focused inquiry,* based on standards of comparison.[2] This inquiry is controlled through the feedback generated by the process of investigation. The collection of data in a specific instance may change focus in response to the collected information. For instance, imagine that you are collecting data to evaluate the appropriateness of

oxygen therapy in your facility over a 4-week period. You initially investigate charts (randomly) to see whether the given therapy is indicated, but you discover that 30 percent of the oxygen therapy is not properly indicated. Now your focus must narrow to that 30-percent group to find the reason for this problem. As you continue to collect and analyze data, feedback from the investigation continues to control the process.

Each RCP is part of the ongoing evaluation process. Whether collecting information, processing data, or improving outcomes as a result of evaluation, every department member is essential to the process. Success depends not only on the physical tasks involved but also on the thinking and caring abilities of the individuals within the organization.

When analyzing information, comparisons with standards must be made. A standard may be a published norm, an ideal result, a common finding in a comparable department, or an established practice. Whatever the case, the standard for comparison must be known, and stated, to ensure that the evaluation is valid.

For an evaluation instrument (the tool used in the collection and/or analysis of data) to be valid, it must measure just what it is intended to measure. For instance, in the oxygen therapy evaluation, the instrument (form) used for the evaluation must in fact reflect the collection and analysis of oxygen therapy orders and the compliance or lack of compliance with appropriate indications. This "use the right tool for the right job" strategy is the essence of *measurement validity*.[3-4]

Another term used to describe evaluation instruments is *reliability*, which refers to the consistency of an evaluation tool.[4] A reliable instrument (usually a check-off form of some type) produces the same results over time. Consider the previous example of the oxygen therapy indications evaluation. A reliable instrument allows collection and analysis of the information to take place in the same manner over the length of the evaluation process, thereby making the process consistent.

⇨ **Thought Prompts**

1. Relate the concept of CT to the evaluation process.
2. Using the oxygen therapy example, create a form (instrument) to allow for valid and reliable measurement of the data.
3. How could you ensure that your instrument is valid and/or reliable?

THE NEED FOR EVALUATION IN RESPIRATORY CARE

In any business environment, evaluation of processes and outcomes is essential. It becomes even more critical when the business involves the care of people. Evaluation is the tool that fosters quality care. Each evaluation involves scrutinizing an organization with the goal of improving the organization's performance in some way. Without an evaluation process in place, the organization simply produces services based on a singular perspective and/or narrow focus. With evaluation the perspective widens, allowing for greater insight, which, in turn, fosters better and safer services. Lack of a solid evaluation system can lead to stagnation, inability, and even danger.

⇨ **Thought Prompt**

4. Describe ways in which an evaluation system could generate excellence in service within an RC department.

TARGET AREAS FOR EVALUATION IN RESPIRATORY CARE

For evaluation to occur, it must have a target or focus. Each evaluation may be focused on one target or may include a combination of targeted areas. The most common *evaluation targets* in the profession of RC are the RCP's performance, the patient or client, the departmental operation or services, and the equipment in use.

Evaluating RCP Performance

In evaluating the RCP's performance, several routes of evaluation exist. There is *self-evaluation* in which the practitioner assesses his or her own performance and judges it accordingly. One might mistakenly view this type of evaluation as low in importance, but the experienced evaluator understands the significance of continuous self-evaluation. Consider that, if all RCPs continuously evaluated their practice and used the evaluative feedback to make improvements, the profession would most likely experience a surge of excellence. Another possible criticism of self-evaluation is that, as humans, we tend to be somewhat lenient on ourselves. The opposing argument claims that we as humans have a huge capacity to be somewhat hard on ourselves, maintaining lofty expectancies and great demands. Somewhere between these two extremes lies the actual outcome of self-evaluation. Using appropriate evaluation tools and standard criteria within the profession, self-evaluation holds much promise for prompting performance improvements.

Another type of evaluation that focuses on the RCP is *peer review*. This is accomplished by either individual or group review or examination of the practitioner's performance. Peer review not only allows the identification of strengths and weaknesses but also permits feedback from peers to foster learning in the form of idea exchanges. Peer review is *not* an opportunity for one practitioner to find fault with another; it should be a chance for healthy exchange and discussion, allowing growth and professionalism to transpire within all participants.

The most common type of evaluation focused on the individual RCP is the *employee performance appraisal*. This evaluation highlights the RCP's critical elements of performance. It is most commonly used in a yearly review schedule and is sometimes linked to salary increases. It is often performed by supervisory personnel and, again, presents an opportunity for feedback on performance. Common performance evaluation categories include:

- Punctuality and attendance
- Application and knowledge of RC tasks
- Interaction and communication
- Professional presentation and appearance
- Use and care of equipment
- Team participation
- Documentation and reporting
- Completion of tasks and time management
- Professional attitude

In the era of total quality management, the performance evaluation (or yearly review) should represent a tool for improving the performance of the RCP through exploration of current practices. Like peer review, the supervisory evaluation should allow both parties to gain insight and it should promote potential. After all, most supervisory personnel within the profession have exhibited some strengths that helped them move into the supervisory role. Why shouldn't this experience be shared with other RCPs in the form of mentoring?

Name: _____John Doe_____

Employee number: _____xxx-xxx_____

Category:	Rating: (1 – 5 with 5 = max.)	Evidence/Criteria:
1. Reveals competence in:		
BLS	5	AHA certificate (copy on file)
ACLS	5	AHA certificate (copy on file)
PALS	____	
NALS	____	
2. Reveals competence in: Basic RC modalities: (List modalities and rate each...)	5	(Evidenced by observation of demonstration)
Advanced RC modalities: (List modalities and rate each...)	5	(Evidenced by observation of demonstration)
3. Reveals competence in compliance with safety standards	5	Score of 80% on interactive assessment program
4. Reveals competence in compliance with infection control standards	5	Score of 80% on post-test after interactive video tutorial
5. Reveals competence in patient assessment skills (List skills...)	5	Observed demonstration and scored 94% on written test
6. Reveals competence in general RC knowledge	5	Credentials: (NBRC) RRT and CRTT
7. Reveals competence in specialty areas	____	(Evidenced by other credentials, such as RPFT or pediatric/perinatal)
8. Reveals competence in patient teaching skills	5	Observed and scored 89% on clinical simulation
9. Reveals competence in leadership ability	5	Organized journal club and held monthly meetings for past 6 months
10. Other (List other evaluated skills, such as protocol use, quality improvement work...)		

Figure 4–1. Example of competency evaluation documentation.

The elements of the performance appraisal are usually rated on a scale, given a score, and then recorded. It is most important to note that the strength of such an evaluation is measured over time. For instance, if, over several years, an employee was rated very highly and then 1 year rated poorly, the evaluation that was "out of sync" with the others would likely be thought of as an exception to the employee's usual practice. Further investigation of both the employee and the supervisor would be indicated to ensure a high level of performance.

Another evaluation model gaining momentum in the field is the *competency evaluation.* This type of evaluation serves many purposes and may be performed as a peer review or supervisory evaluation. It may also be integrated with a performance appraisal (Fig. 4–1). Quite simply put, these checklists outline the important tasks, professional behaviors, and evaluation skills of the RCP. Most educational programs in RC use this type of performance evaluation in clinical practice as part of their curriculum. By using this type of evaluation tool within the profession itself, several objectives are met. First, competence of department staff is en-

sured at a set level. Second, practitioners receive the opportunity to enhance their skills by following the guidelines associated with the competency evaluation. Third, documentation of the competency checkoffs serves as a record of department quality improvement methods, ensuring adherence to recommendations from the Joint Commission on Accreditation of Healthcare Organizations (JCAHO).[5] Figure 4–1 presents an example of a competency checklist document. This type of record is expanded over the span of employment and serves as a cumulative record of an employee's competence in various skills.

The *client survey,* the last type of evaluation pertaining to RCP performance, reflects the patient or client perspective. This type of evaluation consists of collecting data from the patient or client, usually in a checklist format, and rating or ranking the therapist's performance according to the patient or client's view. Very often clients "write in" comments representing some outstanding event, whether it is positive or negative. The following questions are commonly asked during the client survey:

1. Was the service appropriate?
2. Was the service timely?
3. Was the service performed well?
4. Were you treated courteously?
5. Was the service consistent?
6. Were your questions and comments responded to appropriately?
7. Are you satisfied with the service provided?
8. Any comments?

Optimal evaluation concentrates on practitioner skill, professional attitude, and knowledge of the discipline. As you might expect, the best use of these evaluations promotes improvement in the quality of the practitioner's performance. Whatever combination of these evaluation types one may encounter, whether being evaluated or administering the evaluation, one should bear in mind that the purpose is to promote excellence in RC. Cooperation, truth seeking, and communication are primary goals in the process and serve to promote improvements in the delivery of RC services.

⇨ Thought Prompts

5. Consider the evaluations discussed and create a draft of a unified evaluation tool, incorporating all of the evaluations.
6. Discuss the merit of using such an overall system for evaluating practitioners. Also discuss drawbacks.
7. Create a logical argument supporting the use of an overall, integrated evaluation system.
8. How could feedback from such an evaluation system be used to design departmental in-services? Explain.

Evaluating the Patient or Client

The second target category for evaluations is the patient or client. When a patient or client enters into RC service, he or she should be carefully evaluated at several levels. Whereas patient assessment is the collection of data in a given situation, patient evaluation places a value on the collected information and, most important, prompts suggestion for further actions. In evaluating the patient, the practitioner performs assessment and makes a reasonable judgment about the patient's status. Of course, CT is central to any evaluation process and must be practiced continuously to deliver high-quality care.

Patient evaluations are focused on several factors. A concise list of some patient evaluation factors includes:

- The *patient or client condition.* Focus on the state of the patient's health. Is it better or worse than previously?
- The *therapeutic regimen.* Highlight the effect of interventions. Is the treatment effective? Does it produce appropriate responses?

- The *therapeutic response,* or immediate outcome of therapy or services. Is it positive and appropriate?
- The *outcome goals.* Examine the objectives set for a given patient, and weigh their appropriateness and level of achievement. Are the goals reasonable, well matched to the situation, and attainable?
- The *monitoring devices* or *regimens* for the patient. Measure their effectiveness and necessity. Are they sufficient? Indicated?
- The *patient's satisfaction.* Evaluate the patient's subjective level of contentment. Are the services meeting the patient's needs?
- *The overall plan.* Note its pertinence to the case. Is the plan appropriate? Optimal?
- The *overall outcome.* What was the end result? Were the objectives met?

To view the interpretation process, let us examine some examples of patient evaluation in RC.

Situation:	A patient with COPD has just taken an aerosolized bronchodilator treatment.
Assessment:	The patient was experiencing inspiratory and expiratory wheezing throughout both lung fields prior to the treatment. After the treatment, expiratory wheezing is heard over the RUL only. Pulse remained unchanged throughout treatment. Oximetry reading: 93 percent before and 96 percent after treatment. Patient states that "breathing is much better after the treatment."
Evaluation:	The data reveal improvement in *patient condition,* as exemplified by a cessation of inspiratory wheezing and localization of expiratory wheezing to only the RUL and by the increase in oximetry values. Also supporting this evaluation of improvement is the patient's subjective statement of breathing better. No adverse effects are present. The *therapeutic regimen* produced the appropriate *response* of relieving bronchospasm.
Discussion:	The evaluation of this situation includes the interpretation of assessment data (auscultation, pulse monitoring, oximetry reading, subjective response interpretation), the judgment that the patient's condition improved in response to therapy, and the judgment that the therapy was indicated and that the patient's response to it was appropriate. These evaluations represent review of the *process* (situation and its parts), as well as the impact of the treatment (immediate *outcome*). Long-term outcome must be evaluated based on more cumulative (summative) data.

This example focuses on a therapeutic intervention in a patient case. It represents fairly simple data collection and straightforward evaluation of the data. However, the evaluative process is sufficient for this situation.

Evaluating the Departmental Operations

RC departments, whether they exist in acute or subacute rehabilitation or in home care settings, possess a complex variety of services. This variety makes continuous evaluation a "must" for maintaining consistently high-quality service. Examples of departmental evaluations include measurements of time utilization, cost effectiveness, compliance with standards, risk analysis and management, staff competence and preparedness, and customer satisfaction (both internal and external).

Evaluation of *time utilization* measures the allocation and use of the precious resource of time. In a setting in which patient or client care must be carried out on a scheduled basis, some form of evaluation should exist to measure and explain just where time is spent. For instance, measuring the time spent in delivering care in an assigned area and then comparing that time utilization with another assignment may reveal that the assignments are not well balanced. This information may help the department manager to develop improved scheduling patterns. For more information on time management topics, refer to Chapter 6.

Cost effectiveness refers to the cost of a service, procedure, or program weighed against the benefit of such an endeavor. Costs usually associated with RC services include direct costs such as the cost of labor and equipment. Also included are indirect costs such as testing expenses that may be incurred with the service being given. When these costs are outweighed by the benefit or savings of an intervention or service, a positive cost impact exists. On the other hand, when costs exceed savings or benefits, there is a negative cost impact.[6] Numerous tools and formulas exist for measuring cost effectiveness.

Compliance with standards is perhaps one of the most critical areas of evaluation. Each facility is clearly expected to continuously monitor its services and compare them with known standards. For instance, in considering the evaluation of oxygen therapy orders in compliance with indications, the evaluator must use a standard or known indication for criteria. The most widely accepted indications for oxygen therapy are found in the clinical practice guidelines (see App. A) and represent the standard indications for that service.[7]

Risk analysis and management involve measuring the probability of a negative event in the RC process and preventing its occurrence.[8] Any past negative incidents such as patient injury or poor response to an intervention should be analyzed and evaluated to deter the event from recurring. When problems are recognized, policies based on providing improvements are devised. It is imperative that compliance with departmental policy be evaluated as well. Following professional standards, such as the clinical practice guidelines, and monitoring the practice of these standards help to ensure consistent, high-quality care. Instituting RC protocols (standard care plans) and ensuring competence of RCPs also minimize risks, both medically and legally.

Staff competence and preparedness are essential to quality care and warrant serious evaluation. All the evaluations targeted at the RCP (as discussed in the previous section) make up this departmental target. However, when individuals are grouped, often certain trends appear. Noting trends in levels of employee competence or preparedness for certain situations (e.g., cardiac arrest situations) may enable department educational personnel to supply appropriately helpful in-service educational opportunities.

In evaluating *customer satisfaction,* there are two separate perspectives to investigate. First are the external customers, the patients or clients. It is of great importance to measure their satisfaction with the services rendered in order to improve quality (see page 25 for client survey). After all, this is the group that receives the service and should have some input in critiquing it. Second are the internal customers, that is, the employees within an organization. It is also of great importance to measure the degree of satisfaction in this group because this group delivers the service and has control over the delivery of quality care. Employees usually have the best suggestions for improving the processes of an RC department.[9]

Evaluating Equipment Performance and Safety

To form judgments about the proper performance and safety of equipment used in RC requires strict adherence to the equipment assessment guidelines of the manufacturer. If thorough evaluation uses standards of comparison, then those standards must be reviewed and interpreted. There are several sources for finding standards in RC equipment, and many of the organizations are listed in Table 4–1.[10] The JCAHO also documents some safety standards, but the vast majority of guidance comes from the equipment manufacturer, particularly regarding preventive maintenance schedules.

Of great importance in any evaluation of equipment is the analysis of the user. Is the person using the equipment trained appropriately? Is competence ensured? Are there clear and precise procedure guidelines for the use of the equipment? Are the guidelines located in an accessible place? These questions must be answered to thoroughly evaluate equipment use. According to Gibbons,[11] 70 percent of equipment problems are associated with user error.

⇨ **Thought Prompts**

9. Create a short case scenario in which the patient experiences a negative response to therapy. Evaluate the problem. (Be specific, and make a judgment citing evidence and drawing conclusions.)
10. Explain your evaluation of the case.
11. How may this evaluative data be used to improve departmental quality?
12. Examine the elements in a patient survey (page 25).
13. Explain how data from this instrument can prompt quality improvement in RC.

EVALUATION PERSPECTIVES IN RESPIRATORY CARE

Evaluation is performed in a variety of ways and is applied to an array of circumstances in the profession of RC. The most common RC judgments cluster around three main perspectives:

Table 4-1 **ORGANIZATIONS AND STANDARDS FOR EVALUATING RESPIRATORY CARE EQUIPMENT**

American National Standards Institute (ANSI) 1430 Broadway New York, NY 10018	ANSI Z79.2 Tracheal tube connectors and adapters ANSI Z79.3 Oropharyngeal and nasopharyngeal airways ANSI Z79.6 Breathing tubes ANSI Z79.7 Breathing machines for medical use ANSI Z79.9 Humidifiers and nebulizers for medical use ANSI Z79.10 Requirements for oxygen analyzers for monitoring patient breathing mixtures ANSI Z79.13 Oxygen concentrators for medical use ANSI Z79.14 Tracheal tubes ANSI Z79.16 Cuffed orotracheal and nasotracheal tubes
American Society for Testing and Materials (ASTM) 1916 Race Street Philadelphia, PA 19103	F 920 Specification for minimum performance and safety requirements for resuscitators F 965 Specification for rigid laryngoscopes F 927 Specification for pediatric tracheostomy tubes F 984 Specification for cutaneous gas monitoring devices F29.02.01 Cuffed tracheostomy tubes F29.03.01 Standard specification for ventilators intended for critical care F29.03.05 Standard specification for blood gas analyzers F29.03.07 Standard specification for humidifiers F29.03.08 Standard specification for oxygen analyzers for monitoring patient breathing mixtures F29.03.09 Standard specification for electrically powered homecare ventilators F29.03.10 Standard for pulse oximeters
American Association for the Advancement of Medical Instrumentation (AAMI) 1901 North Fort Myer Drive Suite 602 Arlington, VA 22209	AAMI SS-D Spirometers AAMI MIM Guideline for establishing and administering medical instrumentation maintenance programs AAMI SCL Safe current levels for electromedical apparatus
Compressed Gas Association (CGA) 1235 Jefferson Davis Highway Arlington, VA 22202	C-9 Standard color marking of compressed gas cylinders E-7 Standard for flowmeters, pressure reducing regulators G-4 Oxygen G-7 Compressed air for human respiration P-2 Characteristics and safe handling of medical gases V-5 Diameter index safety system
National Committee for Clinical Laboratory Standards 771 E. Lancaster Avenue Villanova, PA 19085	C12 Tentative standard for definitions of quantities and conventions related to blood pH and gas analysis C21 Devices measuring PO_2 and PCO_2 in blood samples C27 Blood gas pre-analytical considerations: specimen collection, calibration, and controls H11 Percutaneous collection of arterial blood for laboratory analysis
National Fire Protection Association (NFPA) Batterymarch Park Quincy, MA 02269	50 Bulk oxygen systems 53 M Fire hazards in oxygen enriched atmospheres 56 B Respiratory therapy 56 H Home use of respiratory therapy 76 B Safe use of electricity in patient care areas 99-1987 Standard for health care facilities
Underwriters Laboratories (UL) 1285 Walt Whitman Road Melville, NY 11747	252 Compressed gas regulators 407 Manifolds for compressed gas

From Hess, D and Kaufman, G: Evaluation, maintenance, and quality control of respiratory care equipment. In: Burton, GG, Hodgkin, JE and Ward, JJ: Respiratory Care: A Guide to Clinical Practice. JB Lippincott, Philadelphia, 1991, p. 112.

the RC *process,* those activities that make up the field of services known as "respiratory care"; the *impact* of the services of RC, represented by the ways in which the patient, client, or community is affected by the service; and the *outcomes* of RC services, the end results of the process[12] (Fig. 4–2). To examine these evaluation perspectives more closely, each will be considered separately. The target areas discussed earlier—the RCP, the patient, the department, and the equipment—are chosen as a result of which perspective the evaluation at hand is directed.

Process Evaluation

Process evaluation monitors the ongoing activities within RC. Process evaluations may focus on the practitioner, the patient, the departmental services, or the equipment in use. It is possible for a department to evaluate its process on a continuous ba-

sis, using several different evaluation instruments. For instance, ongoing process evaluation may include measurement of RCP performance; time utilization; compliance with standards and policies; use and appropriateness of the therapeutic RC plan; and the equipment, assessments, and monitors used. The process of care is evaluated using the targets for focus. These types of evaluations lend insight into the RC process. This allows for improvements to be made on a continuous basis. Remembering that evaluation is feedback-controlled gives clarity to the linkage that exists between evaluation and continuous quality improvement (*CQI*).

Impact Evaluation

Evaluation of the *impact* of RC services is normally focused on the effectiveness of the service in producing a favorable *re-*

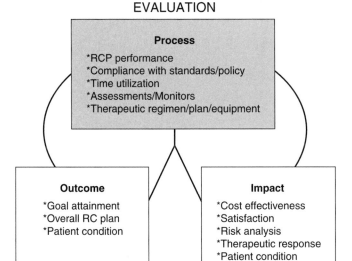

EVALUATION

Process
*RCP performance
*Compliance with standards/policy
*Time utilization
*Assessments/Monitors
*Therapeutic regimen/plan/equipment

Outcome
*Goal attainment
*Overall RC plan
*Patient condition

Impact
*Cost effectiveness
*Satisfaction
*Risk analysis
*Therapeutic response
*Patient condition

Figure 4–2. Concept map of evaluation perspectives.

sponse. Targets commonly examined in an impact evaluation are customer satisfaction, cost effectiveness, risk analysis, and therapeutic response. This type of evaluation is usually performed using data from the patient or client record or department audit reports.

Because it is the responsibility of each practitioner to participate in an ongoing evaluation system, a few precautionary statements are in order. The RCP collecting data for evaluation (as part of the quality improvement process) must use *objective data,* whenever possible, to limit the potential for biasing results. This information should be recorded using standard, nonjudgmental terms and must be used in accordance with appropriate policy guidelines. When data are collected, the results of the impact study should be stated in unbiased, concise, and clear language.

As with process evaluations, impact evaluations can exist in a variety of forms and combinations. They are easily integrated into the day-to-day activities of the RC department and do well in promoting quality improvement and adherence to JCAHO recommendations.

Outcome Evaluation

Outcome evaluation measures the degree to which stated objectives are met, either on a case-by-case basis or in the population as a whole. As opposed to impact, the outcome is associated with more long-term effects. Outcome orientation, focusing primary attention on the end result of a medical service or organization, is presumed to represent a way of examining the total effectiveness of an organization. Considering the magnitude of such an evaluation, it should be obvious that data collection and analysis should be thorough, accurate, and truthful.

When conducting outcome evaluation, the first step is to reflect on the objectives or goals of the original process, person, or object to be evaluated. It is also valuable to use data from

both impact and process evaluations to plan and implement outcome studies. The process is based on feedback and encourages use of the collected information. For instance, to evaluate the outcome of a therapeutic intervention, the investigation must start by examining the objective of the intervention. Then the end result, or outcome, is measured, and a judgment is made regarding the level of success or goal achievement.

These evaluation perspectives should be integral parts of an ongoing evaluation system to ensure positive outcomes and overall success within a department or facility. They are often used in an integrated way so that one (or few) collection instrument(s) may gather information to be applied in many ways (see Fig. 4–2).

Remember that the overall evaluation system should be integrated. Therefore, it is likely that the perspectives of process, impact, and outcome evaluation may overlap. It is also essential to understand that, although department evaluations are an ongoing occurrence, the collected data *must* be analyzed and used, as opposed to collected and simply stored. Again, the evaluation process depends on the CT skills of the RCP for success.

Because evaluations are performed in a timely manner, information is collected in either a formative or a summative manner. This means that some evaluations take place *during* an activity (formative) while other evaluations occur *after* an activity is completed (summative). By definition, a formative evaluation is continuous and feedback controlled, allowing quality to be improved while the process is ongoing. Thus most process evaluations are performed in a formative nature. Conversely, summative evaluations measure the extent to which something has succeeded. Both impact and outcome evaluations serve as examples of summative evaluations.

⇨ **Thought Prompt**

14. Differentiate process, impact, and outcome evaluations.

EVALUATION AND CONTINUOUS QUALITY IMPROVEMENT

Understanding the evaluation process, its targets, and the strategies used to direct evaluations creates the linkage between evaluation and CQI. In fact, the most common purpose for evaluation data in RC is to continuously improve the quality of service. Using feedback from the evaluation process, quality may be improved by examining those areas that are *not* at the desired level of quality and targeting them for changes. These areas are usually termed *indicators,* as they indicate a need for evaluation and effort. Indicators may also be areas of concern, such as those interventions that have associated risks or are numerous in occurrence. Maintenance and readiness of emergency resuscitation supplies may be an area requiring continuous monitoring and evaluation because of its critical nature. Reasons for the lack of quality in any instance may be investigated, and strategies for improvement may be devised. As is evident, the evaluation process should be continuous, ongoing, and useful to the organization.

⇨ Thought Prompts

15. Imagine that you are the department quality improvement leader. Devise and record a plan to improve department quality. Consider creating an overall outline with a timeline or schedule.
16. Who should carry out these quality improvement activities?
17. Provide reasons to institute your quality improvement plan. Refer to these reasons as supporting statements.

OUTCOME MANAGEMENT AND EVALUATION

Managing the outcome of a given situation is facilitated by the evaluation process. To reach a desired outcome, one must set objectives for the outcome, monitor the process, and measure the outcome itself. The entire process grows from the application of information learned from previous and ongoing evaluations.

A simple example of *outcome management* in RC can be generated from our previous oxygen therapy example. When the evaluation revealed that a significant percentage of patients were receiving oxygen therapy without appropriate indication, the objective of decreasing this number was born. Knowing the objective allows plans to be created and followed. In this case, a plan to examine charts to find the source of the problem (Which physicians were ordering therapy inappropriately?) was devised. Once the source of the problem was found, further plans were needed to eliminate the problem. Most commonly, education is the method of choice for correcting a problem like this.

Whether the evaluation process is aimed at a problem or an asset, the outcome may be managed using feedback from the process. To this end, outcome management helps to bring about the desired results, or the *objectives,* of the case. Some common objectives in the outcome management of RC services include shortened length of stay (particularly for ventilator-managed patients), decreased resource use, promotion of cost containment, and improved quality of service.[13]

⇨ Thought Prompts

18. Describe the connection between evaluation and outcome management.
19. Draw a conclusion about the level of participation required of a staff RCP in managing the outcome of a patient on RC services.

Summary

This chapter describes the process of evaluating quality in RC. The specific targets in RC are noted as the RCP; the patient, client, or department; and/or the equipment. The perspectives of evaluation—process, impact, and outcome—are also described and application to RC drawn. The link between evaluation and both CQI and outcome management is discussed.

References

1. Burton, GG and Tietsort, J: Therapist Driven Respiratory Care Protocols: A Practitioner's Guide. Academy Medical Systems, Torrance, CA, 1993.
2. Dignan, M: Program Planning for Health Education and Promotion. Lea & Febiger, Philadelphia, 1992, p. 153.
3. Chatburn, R and Craig K: Fundamentals of Respiratory Care Research. Appleton & Lange, Stamford, CT, 1988, p. 148.
4. Polit, D and Hungler, B: Nursing Research Principles & Methods. JB Lippincott, Philadelphia, 1991, p. 374.
5. Briefings on JCAHO: Special Report 1994. Marblehead, MA, 1993, p. 14.
6. Krieg, AF, Israel, M and Shearer, LK: An approach to cost analysis of clinical laboratory services. Am J Clin Pathol 69:525, 1978.
7. AARC Guideline: Oxygen therapy in the acute care hospital. Respiratory Care 36:1410, 1991.
8. Russel, G: Risky business. Advance for Managers of Respiratory Care 3:29, 1994.
9. Rosenbluth, HG and Peters, DM: The Customer Comes Second. William Morrow, New York, 1992.
10. Hess, D and Kaufman, G: Evaluation, maintenance, and quality control of respiratory care equipment. In: Burton, GG, Hodgkin, JE and Ward, JJ: Respiratory Care: A Guide to Clinical Practice. JB Lippincott, Philadelphia, 1991, p. 111.
11. Gibbons, M: Better safe than sorry. Advance for Managers of Respiratory Care 3:25, 1994.
12. Kettner, P, Moroney, R and Martin, L: Designing & Managing Programs: An Effectiveness Based Approach. Sage Publications, Newbury Park, CA, 1990, p. 196.
13. McCarthy, TP and Kircher, C: The outcome-driven model: A reengineering tool for respiratory care departments. AARC Times 18:49, 1994.

PRACTICE QUESTIONS

1. The components of the evaluation process are:
   I. Regulating and applying data
   II. Forming judgments
   III. Planning
   IV. Reporting and documenting
   V. Analyzing data
   A. I, II, III, IV, and V
   B. I, III, IV, and V
   C. I, II, III, and IV
   D. I, III, and V
   E. II, III, IV, and V

2. Which of the following is *not* a standard in RC?
   A. The clinical practice guidelines
   B. Established past practices
   C. Preliminary results of a research study
   D. ANSI Z79.2

3. *Measurement validity* refers to:
   A. Standard practices
   B. Proven results
   C. Common measurements
   D. Measurement of the intended object

4. *Reliability* refers to:
   A. Proven results
   B. Consistency
   C. Responsibility
   D. Credibility

5. A common target of process evaluation in RC is:
   A. Compliance with standards
   B. Satisfaction
   C. The therapeutic response
   D. Goal attainment

6. A common target of impact evaluation in RC is:
   A. Compliance with standards
   B. Satisfaction
   C. RCP performance
   D. Goal attainment

7. A common target of outcome evaluation in RC is:
   A. Compliance with standards
   B. Equipment
   C. RCP performance
   D. Goal attainment

8. Which of the following describes an *overall* evaluation design for RC?
   A. Incorporates the RCP, the patient, the department, and the equipment as targets
   B. Is used as a source of quality improvement
   C. Is used to decrease departmental direct costs
   D. A and B
   E. A, B, and C

ACTIVITY

Review the following case and list all the areas that may serve as targets for evaluation. Then choose one area and illustrate your plan for evaluating it. Include all components of the evaluation process in your plan.

Your facility is a skilled nursing facility serving the needs of head-injured clients. Twenty RCPs are employed there. You are manager and technical advisor for the RC department. Your scope of services includes oxygen, humidity, aerosol, airway care, and volume expansion therapy, as well as ventilator management, emergency resuscitation, and patient and staff education. Your department works under the direction of a medical advisor, Dr. Woken. She has asked you to devise an RC plan for use in the management of patients who are discharged to their homes. The plan should be flexible and include any required services.

Remember to list the evaluation targets and then create a plan to evaluate one of them. (If you would like to devise the RC plan, go right ahead, or look to Chapter 5 for some help.)

5 | Creating and Modifying the Respiratory Care Plan

Learning Objectives

After reading the chapter and performing the activities within it, the learner will be able to:

- Identify the major components of a respiratory care plan (RC plan).
- Relate the use of clinical practice guidelines in RC to the care planning process.
- Recognize the use of RCP-driven protocols (assess-and-treat care plans) as an important tool in the management of the respiratory patient.
- Recognize the ways in which clinical data are integrated during the formation of an RC plan.
- Recognize the importance of sound CT and high-level assessment skill in preparing the RC plan.
- Correlate treatment indications with therapeutic regimens.

Key Words and Phrases

Assessment	Intervention
Care plan guides	Modifying the plan
Clinical practice guidelines (CPGs)	Monitoring
	PDSA model
Decision tree	Respiratory care plan (RC plan)
Evaluation and regulation	Respiratory care protocols
Identification of problems	
Indications	

THE RESPIRATORY CARE PLAN

To provide quality RC, services must be delivered in a uniform and strategic way. Like all professional services, RC should be deployed based on proven practices and founded on objective evidence. For care to be delivered at a high level of quality, there must be a plan that encompasses the needs of the patient and the interventions to be used. This comprehensive strategy results in the *respiratory care plan* (RC plan), an assessment-based map of service delivery to the pulmonary patient.

Key components of the RC plan include *identification of patient need* (problem), patient *assessment, indication/identification,* creation of *therapeutic objectives, intervention* planning, *monitoring, evaluation, documentation,* and *continuous regulation* of the plan (Table 5–1).

Using the format in Table 5–1 will facilitate the care planning process. There are numerous care planning activities throughout this book, and the learner is advised to use the aforementioned format; however, if another system is in place at a particular facility, that system may be substituted. To focus on the essential planning components, refer to Table 5–2, an example of the recommended format. Keep in mind

when working through the planning process that various elements of the process may be combined. For instance, in the example in Table 5–2, identifying patient need is combined with initial assessment and called "problem identification"; planning interventions and setting objectives are integrated; and the term "recommendations" is substituted for "regulation." These changes in the format are made to promote a flexible approach to the process. It is not the intention of this book to advocate a rigid adherence to one method over another; rather, the intention is to foster solid thinking about the process in order to promote excellence in RC practice.

Table 5–3 does not include the recommendations category. This category is omitted to focus attention on the rest of the care planning process. Making recommendations is highlighted in the section of this chapter called "Critical Thinking as Essential to Creating and Modifying the Care Plan."

RESPIRATORY CARE PLANNING AND THE CLINICAL PRACTICE GUIDELINES

The American Association for Respiratory Care (AARC)[1] *clinical practice guidelines* (CPGs) are "systematically devel-

Table 5–1 **RESPIRATORY CARE PLANNING**

Identification of patient need	Patient enters service either by physician order or existing protocol. Recognize problem requiring RC.
Patient assessment	Perform assessment.
Indication identification	Note indication for intervention (treatment and modality).
Intervention planning	Decide which treatments (interventions) are indicated. Associate therapeutic interventions (treatments or services) with indications and objectives. State frequency and type of intervention. Contingency plans may also be included—that is, if no improvement with one intervention, then another will be instituted. Specify all pertinent information and conditions that exist—such as meds, oxygen concentration. Note resources required such as equipment and personnel.
Therapeutic objectives	State the goals of therapy. Use objective language. Link goals to indications. State objectives in terms of expected outcomes. State what should occur as an outcome of the therapeutic intervention.
Monitoring and assessing	Develop plan for monitoring the patient, as well as the response to interventions. Consider hazards and risks associated with interventions when planning monitors.
Evaluation	Perform evaluation of the patient and the plan on a continuing basis. Perform evaluation as needed (shift, day, week). Perform evaluation when a measurable outcome exists (upon discontinuation of therapy, discharge, or change in condition.) Reevaluate the RC plan at specified intervals—often 24-hr, 48-hr, or 72-hr intervals are used.
Regulation	Use evaluative feedback to make recommendations for changing the regimen.
Documentation	Thoroughly document data to create a medical record of the case and plan.

oped statements to help the practitioner deliver appropriate RC in specific clinical circumstances" (see App. A). These professional tools are a core entity in developing RC plans. They are of particular value in identifying the relationship between clinical interventions and their indications.

Each CPG is formatted in the same manner (Table 5–4). This standardization of format helps the learner to become proficient in understanding the components and content of these guidelines. In every CPG the procedure is defined and identified by name, the setting of the RC practice is identified, the indications for the practice are clearly listed, contraindications are cited, hazards and complications are identified, limitations are discussed relevant to circumstances, the assessments linking the indication to the practice are identified, the outcome assessment criteria are listed, resources are identified, the monitoring plan is advised, frequency of practice is discussed, and infection control is recommended.[1]

⇨ **Thought Prompts**

1. Refer to Appendix A, the AARC clinical practice guidelines, and make a chart listing the indications for incentive spirometry, oxygen therapy in the acute care hospital, and patient ventilator system checks.

2. Correlate these indications to the assessments of outcome in each case.

SYSTEMS FOR CARE PLANNING

A number of systems are used in creating RC plans. These include order and consulting systems that represent outlined methods for care plan guides, and they are often focused on treatment regimens. There are also assessment checklists that assist the care planner in systematically assessing pertinent areas. Flow sheets to list interventions (treatments) and the times they occur are routinely used in RC. Evaluation forms requesting specific information are also part of care planning systems.

These systems and strategies assist the practitioner with keeping records, organizing the plan, and maintaining uniformity in patient care. Such arrangements may also facilitate data entry into computer information systems.

PROTOCOLS FOR CARE PLANNING

RC protocols are models of RC plans that focus on the assessment and treatment of patients. Protocols include all of

Table 5–2 **AN EXAMPLE OF ONE FORMAT FOR RESPIRATORY CARE PLANNING PROCESS**

Problem Identification	Indication of Need for RC Service	Interventions and Objectives	Monitors and Assessments	Evaluations	Recommendations
Diagnosis? Problem?	What specifically will be treated?	What treatment, modality, or method will be used?	What tools/techniques will be used?	What judgments are made?	What next? Changes? Modifications?

Table 5–3 **SOME EXAMPLES OF SIMPLE RESPIRATORY CARE PLANS IN SPECIFIC CASES (NOT INCLUDING HAZARDS, WARNINGS, OR RECOMMENDATIONS)**

Problem	Indications	Interventions and Objectives (Goals)	Monitors and Assessments	Evaluation of Outcome
15-year-old with spinal injury and artificial airway in place	Humidity deficit	Heated aerosol (0.21) to maintain humidity (continuous)	Sputum exam Auscultation	Improved/maintained sputum consistency
	Need to maintain patency of airway	Trach care prn @ least q 24 hr Lung volume expansion and suctioning to maintain sputum clearance and airway patency (prn)	Observe ABG/oxim Pulmonary mechanics Patency of airway check Lab data	Maintain clear BS Improved cough effort Maintained patent airway Reeval plan q 72 hr
	Ineffective cough	Cough training to promote self-care and facilitate weaning from trach (1 training with 1 follow-up evaluation)	CXR VS	
66-year-old with chronic bronchitis (alert and has strong cough)	Bronchospasm (assessed by auscultation and wheezing) Hypoxemia Chronic hypercapnea Dyspnea Yellow sputum production Use of accessory muscles	Provide bronchodilator to reverse bronchospasm (via MDI q 4) Oxygen therapy (0.28) to maintain oxygenation without disturbing ventilatory drive (maintain pH) Obtain sputum for analysis Relaxation and breathing exercises to improve ventilatory efficiency and decrease dyspnea	HR Breathing pattern Oxygen status Vent. status Auscultation Sputum exam Lab data PFTs ECG CXR	Improve: VS BS ABGs Oximetry Values Decrease: Accessory muscle use Bronchospasm Dyspnea Change: Sputum color to white/gray/ or clear Maintain pH Reeval plan q 24 h

ABG = arterial blood gas, BS = breath sounds, CXR = chest x-ray, ECG = electrocardiograph, MDI = metered dose inhaler, Oxim = oximetry, PFT = pulmonary function test, prn = as needed, Reeval = reevaluate, trach = tracheostomy and tube, VS = vital signs.

the components of the care plan and are specifically aimed at a particular problem. They feature a decision tree, which is a graphic representation of the decision process,[2] as a key to selecting interventions. Protocols may be oriented to-

Table 5–4 **FORMAT OF AARC CLINICAL PRACTICE GUIDELINES**

Procedure	Names that procedure is called
Description	Defines and describes the clinical practice
Setting	Where procedure or activity occurs
Indications	Reasons for the activity to occur
Contraindications	Reasons for the activity to not occur
Hazards and complications	Problems that may be associated with the activity and therefore should be watched for
Limitations	Conditions that create restrictions for performing the activity
Assessment of need	Those criteria that represent the indication
Assessment of outcome	Those criteria that represent the end result of the activity
Resources	Equipment, personnel, etc., that are required to implement the clinical activity
Monitoring	Those criteria that require overseeing before, during, and/or after the clinical activity
Frequency	How often the activity should or could occur
Infection control	Risks of infection transfer associated with the activity

ward a modality (e.g., a bronchial hygiene protocol), or they may be oriented toward a patient condition (e.g., pneumonia protocol). Protocols may exist as elements of an overall medical documentation system. Regardless of the orientation, each protocol exists to guide the plan of RC.

The American College of Chest Physicians[3] has prepared a document advocating the practice of RC protocols and describing their value (Fig. 5–1).

Figure 5–2 represents a generic map (flowchart) of the care planning process, while Figure 5–3 may be used as a published model of one organization's approach to the RC planning process.[4] Note the use of graphic illustrations for simplifying the steps within the process. These flowcharts may initially appear confusing, but when one focuses on the sequence that is revealed, the overall organization of the process becomes quite clear. Often, as in Figure 5–2, the shapes used in the drawing have a significant meaning, allowing some differentiation when reading the map. But, as Figure 5–3 reveals, there is sometimes no distinction in shape within the drawing. When attempting to initially "learn" the content of such an illustration, one should first attempt to see the overall picture and then spend time (using practice cases, question-and-answer sessions, or simply discussion) practicing, practicing, practicing.

Physicians have traditionally written orders for respiratory therapy that were specific and allowed no variation by the respiratory care practitioner administering the treatment. If there was a change in patient condition, the physician would be called to have the orders adjusted. However, nationally referenced appropriateness indicators, such as the AARC Clinical Practice Guidelines, have now become widely accepted as practice standards and guides to rational respiratory care. Recently, protocols have been designed to allow assessment by properly trained and credentialed respiratory care practitioners, and for initiation and adjustment of treatment within guidelines previously decided by the physician. In a number of hospitals these protocols have proved highly efficient, safe, and cost-effective. They cover a variety of clinical circumstances including:

A) Perioperative respiratory care
B) Oxygen therapy and titration
C) Ventilator weaning and extubation
D) Bronchial hygiene therapy
E) Pulmonary volume expansion therapy
F) Pulmonary rehabilitation
G) Therapy assessment and prioritization

There are several clear advantages to using protocols (called "assess and treat" protocols in some institutions):

A) Therapy can be adjusted more frequently in response to changes in patient condition.
B) Physicians can still be contacted for major clinical changes, but not minor therapy adjustments, thus reducing nuisance calls.
C) Consistency of treatment can be maintained and nonpulmonary physicians can use appropriate up-to-date methods by simply requesting that protocol therapy be instituted.
D) Respiratory care practitioners become actively involved in achieving the goal of good patient outcome instead of performing rigid tasks. This enhancement of responsibility attracts and retains better educated and qualified practitioners.

Elements of successful Respiratory Care Protocols include:

A) Clearly stated objectives.
B) Outline of the protocol, including a decision tree or algorithm.
C) Description of alternative choices at decision and action points.
D) Description of potential complications and corrections.
E) Description of end-points and decision-points where the physician must be contacted.

Implementation and maintenance of Respiratory Care Protocols require:

A) Use of written protocols with sound scientific basis.
B) Strong medical director support.
C) Intensive education of respiratory care practitioners.
D) Medical staff approval and confidence in the protocol.
E) Frequent auditing of outcomes and continuing education.
F) Adjustment of protocol to meet needs and new scientific evidence.

Figure 5–1. The ACCP position paper on respiratory care protocols. (From ACCP: Respiratory care protocols: Position paper. Chest Oct, 1992, with permission.)

⇨ **Thought Prompts**

3. Define the term "decision tree." Relate this definition to protocol use. How does using a decision tree assist the practitioner in creating care plans?
4. Create a decision tree for using incentive spirometry in postoperative RC.
5. Investigate the various professional protocols in place at your clinical or work facility (e.g., nursing, physical therapy). Compare these with your present understanding of RC protocols.

CRITICAL THINKING AS ESSENTIAL TO CREATING AND MODIFYING THE CARE PLAN

Creating RC plans requires sound CT. RCPs must *identify problems,* question the urgency of the situation, assess the patient, analyze and interpret the data, explain results, and finally regulate the process. At every step in the care planning process, CT is called upon. To practice at a superior level, using RC plans, RCPs must enhance their CT skills by practice and interaction. (See Chap. 2 for information on CT practice strategies.)

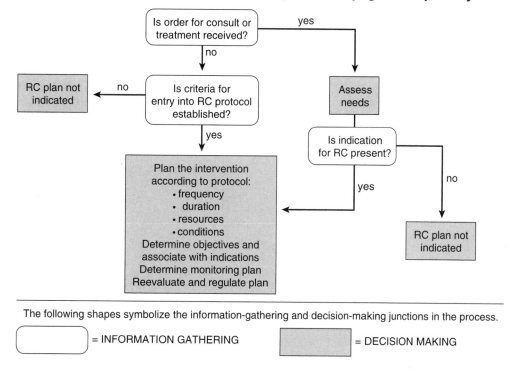

Figure 5–2. A decision tree outlining the respiratory care planning process.

One of the more critical aspects of working with an RC plan is that of *modifying the plan* once it has been implemented. Indications of the need for changing the RC plan include changes in patient conditions, time restrictions, lack of compliance, incorrect initial choices for interventions, poor tailoring of the plan, and/or lack of appropriate indication.

When the patient condition changes, be it for better or worse, the plan must be evaluated to check for appropriateness of interventions. In the case of time restrictions, sometimes plans must be reevaluated and often changed over the course of a set time. For example, incentive spirometry treatments are often administered for a short duration, then stopped and the responsibility handed over to the patient. There are also occasions when the patient refuses or is not able to participate in a particular regimen of care, indicating lack of compliance. In a similar fashion, the initial choice for an RC intervention may be inappropriate in some cases. For instance, a bronchodilator may initially be administered via handheld nebulizer when protocol and cost effectiveness indicate a metered dose inhaler for medication delivery instead. Occasionally an intervention is poorly tailored to an individual, as when a spontaneously breathing patient is placed in the control mode of mechanical ventilation and prevented from spontaneously ventilating. Last, there may be a therapeutic prescription that is not indicated, such as oxygen therapy administration to a patient without hypoxemia or myocardial

problems. In that case, the error must be corrected quickly, tactfully, and efficiently. Many areas within the RC process commonly require adjustments and modifications. For a comprehensive listing of these data, refer to Table 5–5.

Making modifications to the therapeutic regimen *must* be made within the CT realm of being *sensitive to context*. That is to say that each choice for changing or initiating therapy must be considered in light of the total patient care picture. For instance, patient history, a contextual issue, must always be considered in any therapeutic planning endeavor. It would be foolish to call for a stat chest x-ray when auscultation reveals no breath sounds over the chest area of a person who is post-pneumonectomy.

Being sensitive to the context of an issue correlates well with the *Plan-Do-Study-Act* (PDSA) model of investigation formulated by Edward Deming[5] (Fig. 5–4). To make prudent judgments regarding RC planning, one should partake in each element of the PDSA cycle and maintain a continuous pattern of running the cycle. This translates into a continuous evaluate and reevaluate process. It should always be kept in mind that therapeutic plans are part of a continuously changing process; they are not rigid schedules that dictate dogmatic regimens. With these points in mind, the RCP maintains an enlightened, yet open mind during the planning process, always watchful of changes and opportunities as well as careful of hazards and complications.

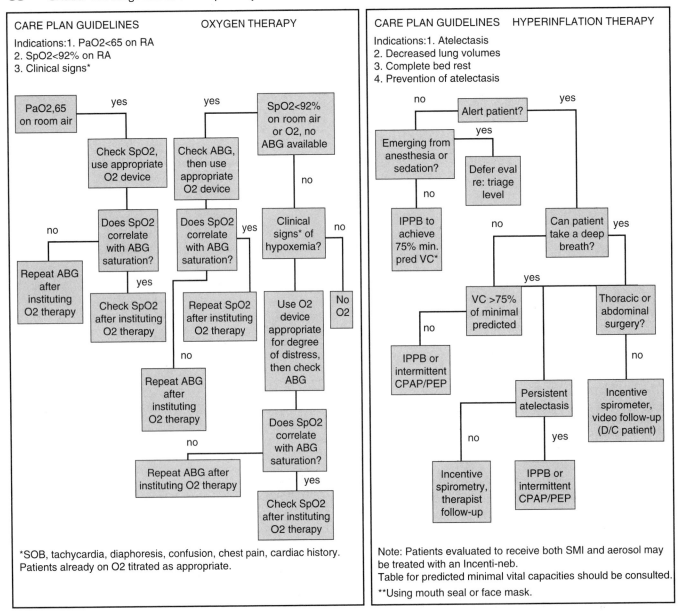

Figure 5–3. Examples of care plan guidelines. (From Stoller, K et al: Physician-ordered respiratory care versus physician-ordered use of a respiratory therapy consult service: Early experience at the Cleveland Clinic Foundation. Respiratory Care 38:1153, 1993, with permission.)

Summary

This chapter reviews the practice of RC planning. Emphasis is placed on the use of strategies and CT as the essential ingredients of RC planning. The clinical practice guidelines from the AARC are suggested as the primary source for guidance in specific clinical instances. Plan modification is cited as a function of CT, and emphasis is placed on the issue of maintaining sensitivity to the context of a situation. The RCP is reminded that practice in the creation of RC plans is important for general practice because it promotes basic skill and facilitates enhanced participation in protocol use.

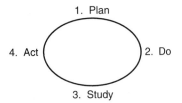

Figure 5–4. The PDSA cycle. (From Deming, E: Out of the crisis by W. Edwards Deming by pemission of MIT and the W. Edwards Deming Institute. Published by MIT, Center for Advanced Educational Services, Cambridge, MA 02139. Copyright 1986 by The W. Edwards Deming Institute.

References

1. Hess, D: AARC clinical practice guidelines. Respiratory Care 36:1398, 1991.
2. Fink, JB: The Respiratory Therapist as Manager. Mosby Yearbook, Philadelphia, 1986, p. 241.
3. ACCP: Respiratory care protocols: Position paper. Chest, October, 1992.
4. Stoller, K et al: Physician-ordered respiratory care vs. physician-ordered use of a respiratory therapy consult service: Early experience at the Cleveland Clinic Foundation. Respiratory Care 38:1153, 1993.
5. Deming, E: Out of the Crisis. MIT Center for Advanced Educational Services, Cambridge, MA, 1986.

Table 5–5 EXAMPLES OF MODIFICATIONS TO THE PLAN

IPPB
  Adjust sensitivity, flow, volume, pressure
  Adjust FIO_2
  Change patient-machine interface (mouthpiece, mask, orotracheal tube)
Incentive breathing devices
  Change type of equipment
  Increase or decrease incentive goals
Aerosol therapy
  Change type of equipment
  Change concentration of medication
  Change dosage of medication
  Adjust temperature of the liquid media
  Modify patient breathing patterns
  Change aerosol output
Oxygen therapy and other gas therapy
  Change mode of administration
  Adjust flow and concentration
  Adjust gas concentration
Chest physiotherapy (bronchopulmonary drainage)
  Alter position of patient
  Alter duration of treatment
  Alter equipment used
  Alter techniques
  Coordinate sequences of therapies
Management of artificial airways
  Change type of humidification equipment
  Initiate suctioning
  Inflate and deflate the cuff
  Alter endotracheal or tracheostomy tube position
  Change endotracheal or tracheostomy tube
  Recommend extubation
Continuous mechanical ventilation
  Adjust ventilator settings
  Change patient breathing circuitry
  Adjust alarm settings
  Institute weaning
  Change weaning procedures
  Change type of ventilator

FIO_2 = fraction of inspired oxygen, IPPB = intermittent positive pressure breathing.
From Barnes, T: The respiratory care plan. In: Barnes, T: Core Textbook of Respiratory Care Practice. Mosby-Year Book, St. Louis, 1994, p 119.

PRACTICE QUESTIONS AND ACTIVITIES

Use the following scenario to practice creating an RC plan. *Note:* As you are creating the RC plan for this patient, take note of the italicized data. They are significant information when planning.

Problem: A 65-year-old woman with a closed head injury is to be discharged to a skilled nursing facility that is a part of your hospital's organization.

As part of your duties you are requested to create the RC plan for this woman. She has a #8.0-mm tracheostomy tube in place. She has been using *21% oxygen* via large-volume heated nebulizer since weaning from mechanical ventilation 3 weeks ago.

Assessments:

$HR = 90$ $PaO_2 = 83\ mm\ Hg\ (on\ 0.21)$

$RR = 14$ $PaCO_2 = 43$

$BP = 110/68$ $pH = 7.36$

$Hct = 43\%$ $HCO_3^- = 24$

Clinical lab data are within normal limits (WNL).

CXR reveals prominent hilar region.

Trach tube is in proper position.

Coarse crackles auscultated bilat.

Sputum is white and frothy in appearance. Produces about 40 mL/day.

Activities of daily living:

Patient is *nonambulatory and requires full assistance for ADLs.* Is *aphasic* and has *poor swallowing* ability. *Does not cough* upon request. *Occasionally responds* to questions with eye movements and blinking.

1. What indications for RC modalities are present in the scenario? (Identify at least two.)

2. List the indicated modalities as well as a suggested frequency and duration if needed. Obtain a copy of the AARC Clinical Practice Guidelines for guidance.

3. State each of these interventions and choose an objective (expected outcome) for each. (If more than one objective is appropriate, report as such.)

4. How will this patient be monitored?

5. How will the objectives be measured? (How will you determine success or failure of the plan?)

6. What events (negative or positive) could signal that a need exists to change the RC plan?

7. Recommend a time interval for the reevaluation of the RC plan.

8. In a concise manner, create the RC plan for this patient.

9. Include a plan for this patient's transport to the other facility.

10. How would the plan differ if (a) the patient's oxygen demand increased? (b) respiratory failure ensued?

6 | Time Management in Respiratory Care Practice

Learning Objectives

After reading the chapter and performing the activities within it, the learner will be able to:

- Clarify the meaning of time management.
- Explain the human problems faced by lack of time structure.
- List the skills involved in time management.
- Relate the concept of time management to RC practice.
- Identify CT as a key to time management.
- Make assumptions based on time analysis.
- Describe the expected outcomes of good time management.

Key Words and Phrases

Effectiveness	Time analysis
Efficiency	Time conflict
Role integration	Time management
Self-discipline	Time structure

TIME MANAGEMENT: WHAT IS IT?

Time management is the process of allocating and lending structure to the events within time. The quantity, quality, and effect of that time use are all important to the health and well-being of an individual or organization. Giving purpose and order to the allocation of time is known as *time structure*. One's perception of his or her time structure is positively correlated with "a sense of purpose in life, self-esteem, reported health, present standing and optimism about the future, and more efficient study habits. Conversely, lack of time structure is related to depression, psychological distress, anxiety, neuroticism, physical symptoms, hopelessness, and anomie."[1] Organizations are merely an extension of the individuals within them, and, when lack of time structure is an individual's problem, the negative impact on that organization is significant.

⇨ Thought Prompts

1. Analyze the concept of time management, and make logical assumptions about its application to the practice of RC.
2. Consider alternatives to good time management. How would your organization or school function if time were *not* carefully structured?
3. What are the human factors associated with time structure?

TIME MANAGEMENT SKILLS

Most of us have practiced time management on some level. Whether organizing study time and materials, arranging supplies for a celebration, or planning a day care arrangement, meticulous attention to timing is crucial. The skills of time management are familiar to all of us, but, like all skills, they require practice and updating.

The most important aspect of becoming a competent time manager is already at your disposal: *CT*. To attempt the management of time, one must *analyze* present time use, *interpret* the analyzed information, *infer* logical strategies for improving time management, and *regulate* appropriately to attain results. Once a method for improving efficiency and/or effectiveness is devised and tried, one needs to *evaluate* the method. This check and recheck system is focal to good time management.

One characteristic that enables both CT and good time management is *self-discipline*. To be self-disciplined is to consistently follow the path that you have mapped out. Although this path will change as you dictate, the changes will be guided by critical thought and will be the result of evaluations made previously. Many successful people have hailed the power of consistent self-discipline as the key to their successes. If not the key, this characteristic is at the very least a doorway to successful practice.

It is also safe to assume that time management is a *systematic* process. To illustrate this systematic process, Figure 6–1 represents a concept map of time management and its associated skills. The primary time management skills are *goal setting, organizing, and regulating the process.*

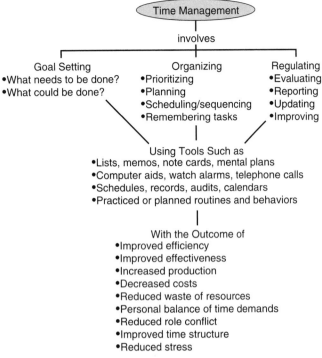

Figure 6–1. Concept map of time mangement.

Setting goals must incorporate a projection of the desired outcome. For instance, a goal that may be common to RCPs is: Improve the time required for emergency department bronchodilator treatments. Reflecting on this goal, we can explore the organizational process as well.

To ensure achievement of our goal, we should investigate both current conditions and potential solutions to barriers. This is part of the planning phase. A key planning resource for time management issues in RC is the *AARC's Uniform Reporting Manual,* which describes common time standards for most RC services. Using the time standards within this manual allows the RCP to analyze and compare time utilization within a department.

Attention to scheduling requirements is essential to ensure the appropriate staffing pattern with consideration to a particular activity. Streamlined systems of documentation featuring checkoffs for assessment, intervention, and outcomes may be extremely helpful in achieving the example goal of reducing the time required for a service. A rating or scoring system for prioritizing or triaging is also helpful (Fig. 6–2).

Prioritizing is a skill that may be acquired through practice (particularly practice in the CT skills) as well as through the consideration of guidelines. For instance, most RC departments have a priority listing that states which of the services is to be given highest priority. Usually, high-priority services include resuscitation and mechanical ventilator troubleshooting; then priorities continue to trend throughout the listing of services. This type of guideline serves as a fundamental base for prioritizing. A routine priority list might look like this[2]:

1. Emergencies
2. Continuous mechanical ventilation
3. Other intensive care services
4. Postoperative care
5. Oxygen administration
6. Prescheduled inpatient basic therapeutics
7. Elective inpatient diagnostic studies
8. Outpatient and ambulatory services

Common sense dictates prioritizing. It should be fairly clear that when two calls are received, an analysis should be made as to which request is more urgent. The ability to conjecture alternatives is of great value. Often several tasks may be combined to decrease required time expenditure and thus improve efficiency. For instance, an RCP who receives a request to initiate oxygen therapy, then immediately receives a request to initiate an aerosolized medication treatment, may gather the equipment required for both therapies and, at the same time, gather information (either over the telephone or from the medical charts) to determine which patient is in greater need. It should also never be forgotten that other medical personnel may be of great assistance when demands increase.

To practice the skills of time management, several tools are used, such as lists, schedules, computer aids, notes, and a wide range of other assistive devices. Most of the tools are memory aids of one kind or another, made to give some cue for the recall of information. However, nothing will substitute for solid CT when time management is at issue. Like all entities involving CT, time management must integrate systematicity with flexibility. This combination of skills allows individuals, particularly RCPs, to enhance strategies for coping with sudden changes in daily schedules. For further illustration of the way that time management concepts are integrated, refer to Figure 6–3.

Because goal setting, prioritizing, and use of tools have been discussed in the preceding paragraphs, the topic of evaluation should be addressed briefly. When evaluating time utilization, the focus is often on efficiency, the workload per cost for a service, or effectiveness, that is, the achievement of the desired outcome. Evaluation of efficiency is easily measured by converting the workload into standard hours (as described in the *AARC Uniform Reporting Manual*) and dividing by the monetary cost of those hours. This standardized figure is then easily compared with previous efficiency as well as with other relative standard data. Effectiveness is evaluated by focusing on the original objective and assessing the level of achievement. It becomes very clear that objectives should be created with their outcome evaluation in mind. For instance, it is much easier to evaluate achievement of the goal of reducing time usage by 10 percent than to evaluate the goal of "improving time management." Specificity in setting objectives lends greater credibility to the evaluation of the effectiveness of achievement of the objective.

The process of evaluation leads to regulation of the process, which continues as the cycle of Plan-Do-Study-Act (see Chap. 5 for more information on the PDSA cycle). In essence, evaluation leads to regulation, which leads to evaluation, which leads to further regulation, and so on.

CCF RESPIRATORY THERAPY EVALUATION

DATE _____

TIME _____

DIAGNOSIS _____ AGE _____

RESPIRATORY THERAPIST _____

ADDRESSOGRAPH

CHART ASSESSMENT

Points	0	x	1	x	2	x	3	x	4	x	Points
Pulmonary History	(-) History (-) Smoking		Smoking history <1 pk a day		Smoking history >1 pk a day		Pulmonary disease		Severe or chronic with exacerbation		
Surgical	No surgery		General surgery		Lower abdominal		Thoracic or upper abdominal		Thoracic with pulmonary disease		
Chest X-ray	Clear or not indicated		Chronic radiographic changes		Infiltrates, atelectasis, or pleural effusions		Infiltrates in more than one lobe		Infiltrate + Atelectasis +/or Pleural effusion		

Lab Test Date _____ WBC ____ Hb ____ Plts ____ | Date _____ | Ph _____ | HCO$_3$ _____ | PaCO$_2$ _____ | PaO$_2$ _____ | Sat/FrO$_2$ _____

PULMONARY FUNCTION TEST
FEV$_1$ _____ FEF$_{25-75}$ _____
FVC _____ PEAK FLOW _____

SpO$_2$ ____ FiO$_2$ ____

Vital Signs HR _____ BP _____ RR _____
TEMP ____ ANTIPYRETIC THERAPY YES ____ NO ____

PATIENT ASSESSMENT

	0	x	1	x	2	x	3	x	4	x	Points
Respiratory Pattern	Regular pattern RR 12–20		Increased RR 20–25		Dyspnea on exertion irregular pattern		Use of accessory muscles. Prolonged expiration or decreased FVC		Severe dyspnea Use of accessory muscles RR>30		
MENTAL STATUS	Alert Oriented Cooperative		Disoriented Follows commands		Obtunded Uncooperative		Obtunded		Comatose		
BREATH SOUNDS	Clear to Auscultation		Decreased unilaterally		Decreased bilaterally		Rales in bases		Wheezing or rhonchi		
COUGH	Strong Spontaneous Nonproductive		Strong Productive		Weak Nonproductive		Weak Productive		No spontaneous cough or may require suctioning		
LEVEL OF ACTIVITY	Ambulatory		Ambulatory with assistance		Nonambulatory		Paraplegic		Quadriplegic		

< or = to 75% of minimal Predicted VC.   Total Points _____

TRIAGE 1 >20	TRIAGE 2 (16–20)	TRIAGE 3 (11–15)	TRIAGE 4 (6–10)	TRIAGE 5 (0–5)

TRIAGE # _____

Figure 6–2. Triage scoring evaluation. (From Stoller, K et al: Physician-ordered respiratory care versus physician-ordered use of a respiratory therapy consult service: Early experience at the Cleveland Clinic Foundation. Respiratory Care 38:1154, 1993, with permission.)

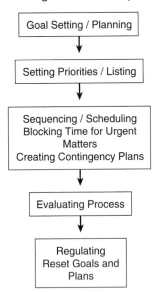

Figure 6–3. Development of a time management scheme.

Thought Prompts

4. Describe the essential skills of time management.
5. Identify time management tools that you use regularly, and discuss their effectiveness.
6. Consider being faced with several patient admissions from an industrial accident. All require RC services. How could you prioritize the needs of these patients? How could you ensure that quality care is delivered to them?
7. Given the example of the need to reduce the time for initiation of aerosolized medication treatments in the emergency department, describe a strategy for evaluating efficiency, as well as a strategy for evaluating effectiveness.

THE SIGNIFICANCE OF TIME MANAGEMENT

In the RC profession, the need for careful time management is critical. To move through the work environment, whether it be in home care, ICU, or any of the other professional areas, the RCP must prioritize duties, schedule events, keep records, carry out the required tasks, and regulate the process. Let us then consider the importance of time management and the consequences of its absence.

Time and its passing have long been a subject of great interest to scientific investigators from many disciplines. The results of some investigations have shed much light on time usage and its effect on us. Rezohazy[3] notes that the shortened workweek (down from an average of 65 to 70 hours), the interest in flexible scheduling, and the general desire for greater control over personal time usage collectively signal the present-day importance of time management. Bond and Feather[1] report lower self-esteem and higher depression rates associated with decreased time structure. And O'Driscoll[4] finds that greater input of time into off-job (personal) activities is related to lower psychological strain, while greater input of time into on-job (work-related) activities is related to higher psychological strain. This is referred to as *time conflict,* when one role, requiring time, interferes with another role.

It is important to note that it is not only interference from "outside" or conflicting sources that creates time conflict; it is the time demands from a single role, such as the busy job of being an RCP, that may create stress. When one is overwhelmed with many duties requiring attention, it is not difficult to see how pressures can build. This pressure often results in dissatisfaction, either with the job or with oneself.

With such high stakes offset by potential gains, one cannot overstate the significance of continuous and careful time management. Our well-being, family life, and work productivity hinge on our potential to balance our time. Time management techniques are used to achieve this balance.

Thought Prompts

8. Examine the conflict created when problems from one area of your life interfere with your time usage in another area.
9. Create a list of possible strategies to prevent time conflict, and discuss each strategy.

ANALYZING TIME USAGE

Analysis of one's time usage involves investigation into the routine processes of daily (work) life. This analysis should include examination of the actual time used for tasks, the outcome of that time, and the general feeling associated with the time spent. In other words, both quantity and quality should be analyzed. Figure 6–4 is an example of a time management self-analysis. Figure 6–5 contains suggested answers to those questions. And Table 6–1 presents "best" answers.

Although this time analysis is based on a managerial scheme, the principles of these practices apply to nonmanagement personnel as well. Certainly, self-management and self-regulation are key elements in the working life of all professional RCPs. Careful analysis of time use enables RCPs to practice safely, competently, and contentedly. It should serve as the initial step in any time management program.

Key factors in time analysis in RC are time savers and time wasters. Most of the tools and general concepts presented in this chapter represent time-saving elements. Some common time wasters in the professional working environment are listed in Table 6–2. These include excessiveness, lack of communication (particularly for delegation purposes), lack of prioritizing skill, lack of motivation, and lack of ability to sequence tasks appropriately.

	Almost Never	Sometimes	Often	Almost Always

1. I keep a written log of how I spend the major portions of my working day.

2. I schedule my least interesting tasks at a time when my energy is at its peak.

3. I review my job and delegate activities that someone else could do just as well.

4. I have time to do what I want to do and what I should do in performing my job.

5. I analyze my job to determine how I can combine or eliminate activities.

6. Actions that lead to short-run objectives take preference over those that might be more important over the long pull.

7. My boss assigns more work than he/she thinks I can handle.

8. I attack short-time tasks (answering the phone, writing notations...) before projects taking a long time.

9. I review the sequence of my job activities and make necessary improvements.

10. I arrange task priorities based on the importance of task goals.

SCORE: _____ _____ _____ _____

Figure 6–4. Time management self analysis. (From Jackson, J: Rationing the scarcest resource: A manager's time. In: Timpe, AD: The Management of Time. Facts on File Publications, NY, 1987, p. 135, with permission.)

Thought Prompts

10. In performing the analysis of time, what assumptions can you make about your time management skill?

11. Which of the "best" answers do *not* fit into the role of the RCP as you see it?

THE OUTCOMES OF TIME MANAGEMENT PRACTICES

The positive results of sound time management practices for the RCP are abundant. One extremely important outcome is that of minimizing stress. If careful time management can help to alleviate sources of personal and professional stress, there seems to be no possible argument for *not* employing time management principles in both job and nonjob areas. Higher self-esteem, lower depression rates, and a more positive outlook on the future are correlated with well-developed time structure.[1]

On a more concrete level, time management practices can improve *efficiency,* particularly by eliminating wasted time. One often hears busy professionals express concerns over their lack of time. There is no doubt that time is a most precious resource. When this resource is "saved" and efficiency improved, then job satisfaction, productivity, and general *ef-* *fectiveness* are all enhanced positively. When it is "wasted," a great loss occurs.

It should be remembered that efficiency and effectiveness are sometimes at odds with one another. Consider the situation of patient education. There are times when patient education requires more than the average time allotment to achieve effectiveness (likely because of patient learning needs), at a cost

Item analysis for scoring time analysis:
Check your answers and note the score of each.

Item	Almost Never	Sometimes	Often	Almost Always
1.	2	3	2	1
2.	0	1	2	3
3.	0	1	2	3
4.	0	1	2	3
5.	2	3	2	1
6.	2	3	2	1
7.	3	2	1	0
8.	3	2	1	0
9.	1	2	3	2
10.	0	1	2	3

Score analysis:
>25 Efficient use of time   <15 Ineffective time management

Figure 6–5. Suggested time analysis answers. (From Jackson, J: Rationing the scarcest resource: A manager's time. In: Timpe, AD: The Management of Time. Facts on File Publications, NY, 1987, p. 135, with permission.)

Table 6–1 BEST ANSWERS TO TIME ANALYSIS QUESTIONS

1. Sometimes, recording time usage is a useful task but not a continuously needed one—constant recording wastes time.
2. Almost always, self-discipline will be rewarded when tasks are accomplished in a timely fashion—get the "scut" out of the way first.
3. Almost always, doing what you should do is imperative, but, if someone else is in a better position to do it, delegate if possible.
4. Almost always. If good time management is in place, this should occur as a result.
5. Sometimes, constant analysis like continuous recording may become a time waster instead of a time saver.
6. Sometimes, one cannot always answer to the short-term needs; sometimes the long-range plan must be addressed without "other" things coming first.
7. Almost never. This type of dilemma may result from poor supervision or lack of production on the part of the worker.
8. Almost never. From a managerial standpoint this is ineffective, but when the short-time tasks are part of an assignment, they must be addressed efficiently.
9. Often, this action promotes continuous improvement and optimizes efficiency.
10. Almost always, this is a must for sound time managers.

From Jackson, J: Rationing the scarcest resource: A manager's time. In Timpe, AD: The Management of Time. Facts on File Publications, NY, 1987, with permission.

Table 6–2 TIME WASTERS IN RESPIRATORY CARE

Excessiveness (trying to accomplish too much/unreasonable expectations)
Lack of communication
Lack of prioritizing skill
Lack of motivation
Lack of ability in sequencing routine tasks

equivalent to efficiency. It would clearly be unwise to force a standard time allotment onto an individual condition in which lack of achieving *effect* might increase patient risk.

⇨ Thought Prompts

12. Examine the potential outcomes of time management, and express an argument supporting its use.
13. How does time management affect an organization? An individual?

Summary

Time management is defined as the allocation and control of time. It is related to time structure, the organization of time. Stress reduction is cited as the most significant reason for using time management. CT is noted as the foundation of time management. Self-discipline is a primary characteristic needed for proficient time management. The key ingredients of time management are goal setting, organizing, and regulating. Important tools of time management are lists, schedules, calendars, and other organizers and/or cues.

Time analysis is suggested as the first step in the time management process. It is part of the planning stage. The outcomes of time management include improved efficiency, improved effectiveness, and reduced stress.

References

1. Bond, MJ and Feather, NT: Some correlates of structure and purpose in the use of time. Journal of Personality and Social Psychology 55:327, 1988.
2. McDonald, PM and Mathias, JH. In Scanlan, CL: Egan's Fundamentals of Respiratory Care, ed 6. Mosby, St. Louis, 1995, p. 22.
3. Rezohazy, R: Recent social developments and changes in attitudes to time. International Social Science Journal 107, 1986.
4. O'Driscoll, M et al: Time devoted to job and off-job activities, interrole conflict, and affective experiences. Journal of Applied Psychology 77:277, 1992.

PRACTICE QUESTIONS

1. To improve efficiency, which of the following tasks should be performed first when starting a time management program?
   A. Listing tasks to be done
   B. Organizing evaluation data
   C. Creating a scheduling system
   D. Performing a time analysis
   E. Gathering tools for time management practice

2. All of the following statements are true of time management except:
   A. It is the process of allocating and structuring the events within time.
   B. Its practice is closely related to the CT process.
   C. It is synonymous with *efficiency*.
   D. Its practice may improve job satisfaction.

3. In performing a time analysis, all of the following would be reviewed except:
   A. Clinical competence
   B. Sequencing of tasks
   C. Prioritizing ability
   D. Resource use
   E. Reporting (documenting of time use)

4. Which of the following would most likely occur first in the case of sudden unemployment?
   A. Lack of CT
   B. Lack of time structure
   C. Loss of self-discipline
   D. Lack of time management practice

5. In which of the following instances would efficiency take precedence over effectiveness?
   A. General patient care
   B. Ventilator management
   C. Patient education
   D. Equipment storage
   E. Documentation

6. Which of the following is not viewed as something that should be done almost always?
   A. Attend to short time tasks before projects that take longer.
   B. Prioritize according to the importance of a task.
   C. Delegate when appropriate.

D. Attack least interesting things when at peak energy level.

E. Have time for doing enjoyable as well as necessary job functions.

7. The most likely priority listing of the following would be:
   I. Outpatient care
   II. Continuous mechanical ventilation
   III. Oxygen administration
   IV. Elective inpatient diagnostic studies
   V. Emergency care
      A. I, II, III, IV, and V
      B. V, IV, III, II, and I
      C. V, II, III, IV, and I
      D. II, V, III, IV, and I
      E. III, V, II, I, and IV

8. Examples of time conflict in the RC profession would include all of the following except:
   A. Attending to telephone requests while conducting a staff meeting
   B. Changing the sequence of a daily schedule to accommodate a new patient
   C. Remaining at work late to complete a transport service on the evening of a family gathering
   D. Having simultaneous requests to respond to urgent situations
   E. Performing a home care evaluation in the allotted time allowance but requiring more time to perform documentation of the evaluation

9–11. Match the term in column I with the appropriate phrase in column II:

I	II
9. Time management	A. Ordered arrangement of time
10. Time structure	B. Created by role interference
11. Time conflict	C. Has the outcome of improved effectiveness

ACTIVITIES

1. Imagine that your place of employment has determined that a program aimed at conserving the resource of time be implemented. You have been asked to join the committee for designing the program. What suggestions do you have? What is the best first step in such a program? (Record your suggestions.)

2. Once you have created an outline of your program, begin discussion with fellow students or coworkers. Be sure to have reasonable evidence to support your choices, and be willing to incorporate other ideas as well.

3. Perform the time analysis on page 45. Evaluate your results and pinpoint weaknesses. Make inferences as to how you might improve your time management practices.

An Introduction to the Case Studies

The following chapters represent a series of case studies featuring several disease states and common modalities used in the care of those suffering from them. The objective of this book is to allow for exploration of thought as well as for development of understanding. The cases follow a developmental strategy, beginning with John Tie, a basic postoperative patient, and progressing to Kyle Hicks, a critically ill neonate requiring major intervention.

The "Thought Prompts" follow sections of the case. Your active participation is advised at these junctures. It is also suggested that you initiate discussion focusing on the case problems. To assist you in the learning process, you should use a wide variety of resources, namely, your own knowledge (particularly your common sense); your classmates and peers' experience and knowledge; your instructor, mentor, or tutor; the appendixes within this book; and suggested books and journals, as well as any other resource available to you. Your instructor should serve as a guide in your study. At times, particular emphasis may be desired by an instructor. This may take the form of selecting some thought prompts for practice, while leaving others for a later time. I have not found this approach to be detrimental when I have tried it with students. Content coverage is often a function of time management. The cases allow for flexible and collaborative activity. Enjoy!

7 | John Tie: A Postoperative Patient with Lobectomy

Learning Objectives

After reading the chapter and performing the activities within it, the learner will be able to:

- Differentiate among critical, noncritical, and useful assessment data.
- Identify relationships between disease and/or problem states and assessment findings.
- List indications for oxygen therapy, arterial blood gas sampling, pulse oximetry, and hyperinflation therapies.
- Determine the therapeutic objectives for the modalities.
- Outline and modify the respiratory care plan (RC plan).
- Evaluate patient responses.
- Conjecture alternatives and make recommendations regarding the RC plan.
- Evaluate the outcome of the interventions.

Key Words and Phrases

Aerosol administration
Arterial blood gas
  (ABG) sampling
Assessments
Atelectasis
Bronchial adenoma
Incentive spirometry
Indications

Intermittent positive pressure
  breathing (IPPB)
Oxygen therapy
Patient therapeutic responses
Preventive measures
Pulse oximetry
RC plan
Risk factors

INTRODUCTION

This case presentation follows the clinical course of a male patient, John Tie. The case is reported as concisely as possible. Certain information is omitted to maintain brevity as well as to promote problem solving.

HISTORY OF CURRENT ILLNESS

Mr. John Tie is a 32-year-old man who was admitted to this institution for open lung biopsy and evaluation. His history includes 6 weeks of progressive dyspnea and a chest radiograph (taken during the second week) revealing a 1-cm-diameter density in the right upper lobe (RUL). A diffuse reticular pattern was observed at the periphery of the density. Mr. Tie has been afebrile and without pain. His other primary complaint is that of a persistent dry cough, which occasionally produces blood-tinged sputum.

PAST MEDICAL HISTORY (PMH)

Aside from the recent events noted, his history is noncontributory. Mr. Tie maintains regular physical examination visits with his primary physician.

SOCIAL HISTORY

Married with two healthy children. Occasional alcohol intake, described as a "weekend beer or two." Has smoked two packs of cigarettes a day for 18 years. Is still smoking. Plays basketball weekly and takes 2-mile walks daily.

EMPLOYMENT HISTORY

Employed full time as an accountant. Has worked for his present employer for 8 years. Had previously worked as a grocery clerk.

PHYSICAL EXAMINATION

HR (heart rate) = 104.
Pulses are bounding.
BP (blood pressure) = 125/90 mm Hg.
RR (respiratory rate) = 22.
Ht. (height) = 75 in.
Wt. (weight) = 190 lb.
Auscultation reveals coarse crackles and expiratory wheezing over the right lung. Otherwise clear breath sounds (BS). No abnormalities observed through palpation or percussion. Normal neurological examination. Otherwise, physical examination is negative for unusual findings.

APPEARANCE

Mr. Tie presents with obvious shortness of breath (SOB) and marked use of accessory muscles. He is well nourished with no other apparent physical limitations. He is alert and oriented. There are no visible scars or lesions on the body. He presents as a dyspneic and anxious, although pleasant, person.

ADMITTING DIAGNOSTICS

Labs: RBC = $4.9 \times 10^6/mm^3$
HB (hemoglobin) = 14.5 g/dL
Hct (hematocrit) = 50%
WBC (white blood cell count) = $6600/mm^3$
DIFFERENTIAL:
Segmented neutrophils: 50%
Bands: 6%
Eosinophils: 5%
Basophils: 1%
Lymphocytes: 30%
Monocytes: 8%
ABG:
PaO_2 = 85 mm Hg
$PaCO_2$ = 41 mm Hg
pH = 7.39
SaO_2 = 94%
ECG: Normal sinus rhythm with HR = 104 bpm
PFT:
FVC = 80% of predicted
FEV_1 = 80% of predicted
$FEF_{25\%-75\%}$ = 84% of predicted
Predicted postoperative FEV_1 = 3 L/min

➪ Thought Prompts

1. Are any *risk factors* identified in the admission note?
2. If so, list them and describe the risks.

3. If there are significant risk factors, how do they relate to the patient's expected course of treatment and eventual outcome?
4. What problems could arise in this case, based on what you have discovered?
5. Are there any *preventive measures* that should be planned at this point?

SURGICAL NOTATIONS

Anesthesia Service Excerpt

Orally intubated with #9.0-mm endotracheal tube.
Anesthesia in use for 2 h without adverse signs or symptoms.
Vital signs remained stable and within normal limits throughout procedure.
Fluids maintained and monitored.

Surgical Service Excerpt

Procedure: RUL lobectomy
The 1-cm nodule was observed and excised, along with surrounding lobar tissue. Prepared and sent to pathology for examination.
No problems occurred intraoperatively.
Incision closed with minimal bleeding. Operative time: 2 h.

Pathology Service Excerpt

The 1-cm mass removed from the RUL of this 32-year-old man is determined to be a *bronchial adenoma*. Vascular involvement throughout the lobe.

➪ Thought Prompts

6. Do any of the *assessment* findings recorded in the surgical notations indicate a poor response to the surgical procedure?
7. List some of the immediate postoperative problems that could arise.
8. How could the *RC plan* address these possible risks?
9. What is bronchial adenoma and what are its associated problems?

NURSING NOTATIONS

Nursing Diagnoses

- Pain, acute: related to surgical procedure
- Breathing pattern, ineffective: related to fatigue and pain
- Gas exchange, impaired: related to thoracotomy
- Activity intolerance: related to acute pain

Patient Outcomes

- Patient verbalizes comfort.
- Patient demonstrates effective breathing pattern.
- ABGs are within normal limits.
- Patient verbalizes increased comfort during activities.

RESPIRATORY CARE PLAN

In accordance with physician orders.

Indications for Service

1. Potential for development of *atelectasis*
2. Short-term oxygen and humidity requirement
3. Potential for $\dot{V}/\dot{Q}$ imbalance, related to thoracic surgery

Therapeutic Objectives

1. Prevent the development of atelectasis.
2. Maintain PaO_2 between 80 and 100 mm Hg.
3. Prevent postextubation tracheal edema.
4. Prevent secretion retention.
5. Assess and document oxygenation and ventilation status, according to patient condition, using *ABG sampling* and/or *pulse oximetry*.

Interventions

1. *Incentive spirometry* q 1 h (initial treatments by RCP with subsequent treatments monitored by nurse and patient).
2. *Oxygen therapy* via nebulizer postoperatively, titrated to achieve objective PaO_2 range of 80 to 100 mm Hg. Discontinue when ABGs are within normal limits and patient demonstrates spontaneous coughing ability.
3. Reassess and evaluate plan q 24 h, unless patient condition indicates change in plan.

Diagnostics and Monitors

1. Postoperative ABG and prn sampling in response to clinical signs of deteriorating oxygenation and/or ventilation.
2. Pulse oximetry continuously during postanesthesia period, then prn.
3. Reassess and document prn.

⇨ **Thought Prompts**

10. List the RC modalities to be implemented. After each, record the assessments to be used in evaluating the *therapeutic response* (and eventually the outcome of the objectives).

11. List probable patient responses to support that the therapeutic objectives *were achieved.*
12. List patient responses to indicate that the objectives of therapy were *not* met.
13. Is the care plan complete and appropriate?
14. Do you have anything to add to it?

Clinical Notations

Information not recorded may be considered normal or insignificant. All interventions are in accordance with physician order.

General Care	RC Assessments	RC Interventions	Recommendations
Preop: IV access. Antibiotics initiated.	Dyspnea noted Nodular density in RUL confirmed HR = 110; RR = 22 Predicted IC = 2.7 L Actual IC = 2.4 L PaO_2 = 70 on 21% O_2	Preop teaching of IS	Early postoperative evaluation and intervention
Day 1	RUL lobectomy Alert in post-operative care unit R side chest tube attached to drainage unit 400 mL bloody drainage from chest tube Weak, nonproductive cough HR = 116 PaO_2 = 75 on 40% O_2 SpO_2 = 94% IC = 1.8 L CXR clear C/O pain over R chest and shoulder	Cough and DB and IS q 1 h O_2 via neb @ 40%	
Day 2	Temp = 38.5°C < 100 mL drainage from drainage unit Weak, congested cough PaO_2 = 73 on 50% O_2 SpO_2 = 93% Patchy atelectasis in RLL HR = 129 (sinus) IC = 1.5 L Suction to chest drainage unit d/c'd	IS continues/q 1 h O_2 via neb @ 50%	
Day 3	Temp = 39°C PaO_2 = 80 on 50% O_2 SpO_2 = 95% HR = 115 IC = 1.8 L	IPPB q 3 h	
Day 4	Temp = 37°C PaO_2 = 82 on 45% O_2 SpO_2 = 95% Clearing of CXR IC = 2.0 L Chest tube removed	IPPB q 4 h O_2 @ 0.45	
Day 5	PaO_2 = 82 on 35% O_2 Clear CXR HR = 98 SpO_2 = 97% IC = 2.3 L	O_2 @ 0.35 IPPB d/c'd	
Day 6	PaO_2 = 89 on 21% O_2 Discharge planned		

C/O: complains of, CXR: chest x-ray, DB: deep breathing, d/c'd: discontinued, IC: inspiratory capacity, IPPB: intermittent positive pressure breathing, IS: incentive spirometry, neb: nebulizer, R: right, pressure breathing, RLL: right lower lobe, RUL: right upper lobe.

⇨ **Thought Prompts**

15. What indicated the need to change to *intermittent positive pressure breathing (IPPB)* on Day 3?
16. Is this modification in therapy appropriate?
17. Record a description of a complete IPPB order. Include as much detail as needed.
18. What would the therapeutic objective be at this point?
19. How would the outcome of therapy be evaluated?
20. Explain the regulation of oxygen therapy in this case. Was it appropriate? What assessments were used to guide the therapy?

Refer to Figure 7–1 for an overview of the pathogenesis of atelectasis. Figure 7–2 illustrates the integration of RC plan components. Note that the basic elements are assessments, monitors, interventions, and outcomes. Notice that this scheme resembles the basic RC planning process.

Bibliography

AARC: Clinical practice guideline: Incentive spirometry. Respiratory Care 36, 1991.

AARC: Clinical practice guideline: Bland aerosol administration. Respiratory Care 38, 1993.

AARC: Clinical practice guideline: Oxygen therapy in the acute care hospital. Respiratory Care 36, 1991.

AARC: Clinical practice guideline: Arterial blood gas sampling. Respiratory Care 37, 1992.

AARC: Clinical practice guideline: Pulse oximetry. Respiratory Care 36, 1991.

AARC: Clinical practice guideline: Intermittent positive pressure breathing. Respiratory Care 38, 1993.

DesJardins, T: Clinical Manifestations of Respiratory Disease, ed 3. Mosby-Year Book, St. Louis, 1995.

Farzan, S: A Concise Handbook of Respiratory Diseases, ed 3. Appleton & Lange, Stamford, CT, 1992.

Kacmarek, R and Pierson, D: Foundations of Respiratory Care. Churchill Livingstone, New York, 1992.

Miller, A: Pulmonary Function Tests. Grune & Stratton, Orlando, 1987.

Ruppel, G: Manual of Pulmonary Function Testing. Mosby, St. Louis, 1994.

Scanlan, C, Spearman, C and Sheldon, R: Egan's Fundamentals of Respiratory Care, ed 6. Mosby, St. Louis, 1995.

Wilkins, RL and Dexter, JR: Respiratory Disease: A Case Study Approach to Patient Care, ed 2. FA Davis, Philadelphia, 1997.

PRACTICE QUESTIONS

1. Which of the following clinical conditions is an indication for incentive spirometry?

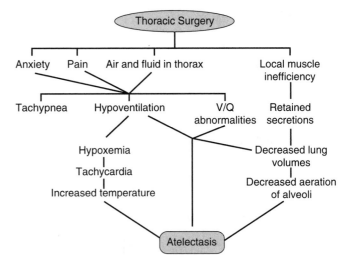

Figure 7–1. Pathogenesis of postoperative atelectasis. (Note the relationships rather than cause and effect.)

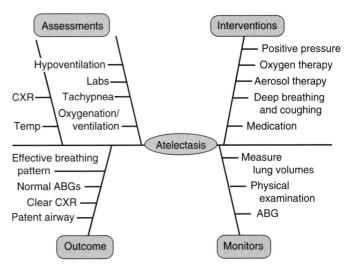

Figure 7–2. Integrated components of the RC plan in this case.

A. Hypoxemia
B. Atelectasis
C. Thoracic or upper abdominal surgery
D. A and B
E. B and C

2. The volume of air that the patient inspires when performing incentive spirometry should approximate:
A. FVC
B. IC
C. FRC
D. TLC
E. V_t

3. All of the following contribute to the development of atelectasis except:
A. Respiratory muscle insufficiency
B. Retained secretions
C. Hypoventilation
D. Hypoxemia

4. Which of the following are indications for oxygen therapy?
   I. Hyperventilation
   II. Hypoxemia
   III. Postanesthesia recovery
   IV. Acute myocardial infarct
   V. Lung cancer
      A. I, II, and III
      B. I, II, and IV
      C. II, III, and IV
      D. I, III, and V
      E. II, III, and V

5. IPPB is indicated in all of the following situations except:
   A. Inability to clear secretions
   B. Atelectasis that does not respond to other therapies
   C. Short-term ventilation
   D. Aerosol delivery when muscle fatigue is present
   E. Tracheoesophageal fistula

6. Which of the following are clinical signs of atelectasis?
   A. Increased temperature
   B. Patchy markings on CXR
   C. Tracheal shift toward the affected area
   D. Elevated diaphragm
   E. All are signs of atelectasis

7. Which of the following are therapeutic objectives of oxygen therapy?
   I. Maintain normoxia.
   II. Decrease myocardial work.
   III. Stabilize acid-base balance.
   IV. Provide enriched oxygen environment for increased metabolic needs associated with severe trauma.
   V. Provide premature infant with PaO_2 of 90 to 100 mm Hg.
      A. I, II, and III
      B. I, II, and IV
      C. II, III, and IV
      D. I and V
      E. I, III, and IV

8. The optimal patient response to treatment with incentive spirometry would be the following:
   A. Chest radiograph is negative for atelectasis.
   B. Patient verbalizes no difficulty breathing.
   C. Cough is nonproductive.
   D. Patient is discharged from the hospital.
   E. No signs of respiratory compromise are observed on physical inspection.

9. The most reliable indicator that a patient understands the maneuver for incentive spirometry is:
   A. He can explain the procedure.
   B. He documents that he has learned the procedure.
   C. He demonstrates the procedure.
   D. He verbalizes understanding.
   E. His spouse assures the RCP that the patient understands.

10. All of the following are indications for aerosol therapy except:
   A. History of hyperresponsive airways
   B. Upper airway edema
   C. Sputum induction
   D. Postextubation edema
   E. Bypass of the upper airway

ACTIVITIES

1. Complete the table below by listing the assessments used in this case and assigning them the value of critical, useful, or nonessential information.

ASSESSMENTS		
Critical	Useful	Noncritical
Preoperative		
Intraoperative		
Postoperative		

2. Relate the care plan used in this case to other situations. What other surgical conditions may indicate the use of such modalities as incentive spirometry?

3. Research the pulmonary function measurements described in the preoperative assessment. What is he significance of comparing values to predicted values?

4. Develop a teaching plan for a patient such as Mr. Tie. Your objective will be to ensure his or her understanding of the purpose and practice of incentive spirometry.

8 | Kate Wind: A Pediatric Asthma Patient

Learning Objectives

After reading the chapter and performing the activities within it, the learner will be able to:

- Identify assessment data associated with asthma.
- Relate therapeutic objectives to their options.
- Identify monitoring strategies for evaluating asthma severity and therapeutic response.
- Identify current protocols for asthma management.
- Recognize educational strategies for promoting asthma self-management in patients.

Key Words and Phrases

Albuterol
Asthma
Bronchodilators
Discharge planning
Nebulizer
Oximetry
Oxygen (O_2) therapy

Patient education
Peak expiratory flow rate (PEFR)
Pulsus paradoxus
Steroids
Therapeutic response

INTRODUCTION

This case highlights the events surrounding a 9-year-old girl with *asthma*. The care plan should follow the "Guidelines for the Diagnosis and Management of Asthma" (Fig. 8–1). Remember, some details have been omitted for brevity and/or to facilitate problem solving.

RESPIRATORY CARE NOTE

9:15 AM Emergency Department.

A 9-year-old girl is admitted to the emergency department with the diagnosis of asthma. This patient has had one prior admission for asthma at this facility, according to the admission record. On physical examination the following are noted:

Patient complains of shortness of breath, chest "tightness," and feeling "very tired." States taking 2 Proventil "inhaler" treatments over last hour at home.
Has had cold symptoms for 2 days.
Dyspnea evidenced by marked use of accessory muscles for breathing.
HR is 148.
RR is 38.
BP is 110\68.

Pulsus paradoxus of 20 mm Hg noted.
Is afebrile.
Decreased BS with distant *inspiratory and expiratory* (I&E) wheezing.
Percussion note is hyperresonant.
Dry cough.
Peak expiratory flow rate (PEFR) is 162 L/min.
Baseline predicted PEFR is 270 L/min.
(Current PEFR of 162 is 60 percent of this predicted.)
Oxygen saturation (via *oximetry*) is 90 percent.
ABG pending.
Face is flushed over cheeks.
Dark circles noted under eyes.
Is diaphoretic.
Some trembling of the hands noted.
CBC pending.
Allergic to several strains of pollen.
States not eating or drinking anything since last evening.

HISTORY (OBTAINED FROM PATIENT AND MOTHER)

Diagnosed with asthma about 2 years ago, when seasonal "hay fever" seemed to become more severe. Has used Proventil MDI prn since. States using MDI infrequently except during early spring.

Chart 12

Acute Exacerbations of Asthma in Children
*Emergency Department Management**

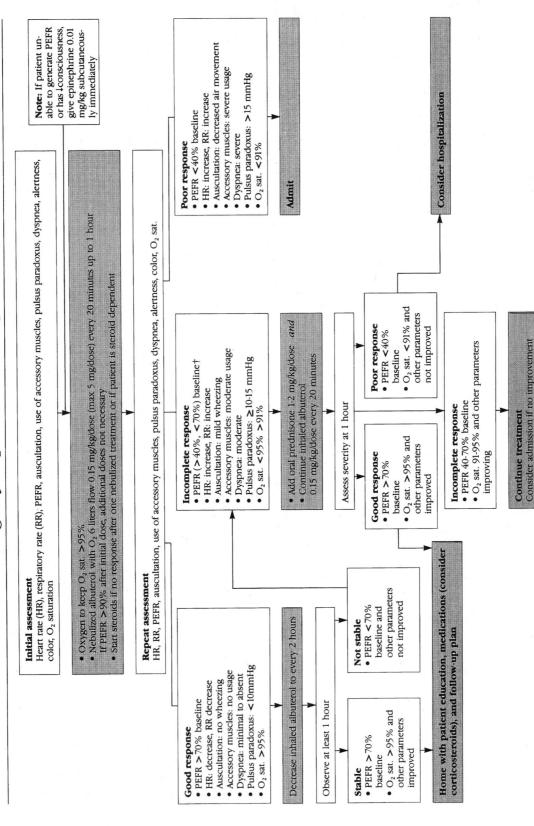

Initial assessment
Heart rate (HR), respiratory rate (RR), PEFR, auscultation, use of accessory muscles, pulsus paradoxus, dyspnea, alertness, color, O_2 saturation

- Oxygen to keep O_2 sat. >95%
- Nebulized albuterol with O_2 6 liters flow 0.15 mg/kg/dose (max 5 mg/dose) every 20 minutes up to 1 hour
- If PEFR >90% after initial dose, additional doses not necessary
- Start steroids if no response after one nebulized treatment or if patient is steroid dependent

Note: If patient unable to generate PEFR or has ↓consciousness, give epinephrine 0.01 mg/kg subcutaneously immediately

Repeat assessment
HR, RR, PEFR, auscultation, use of accessory muscles, pulsus paradoxus, dyspnea, alertness, color, O_2 sat.

Good response
- PEFR >70% baseline
- HR: decrease, RR decrease
- Auscultation: no wheezing
- Accessory muscles: no usage
- Dyspnea: minimal to absent
- Pulsus paradoxus: <10mmHg
- O_2 sat. >95%.

Incomplete response
- PEFR (>40%, <70%) baseline†
- HR: increase, RR: increase
- Auscultation: mild wheezing
- Accessory muscles: moderate usage
- Dyspnea: moderate
- Pulsus paradoxus: ≧10-15 mmHg
- O_2 sat. <95% >91%

Poor response
- PEFR <40% baseline
- HR: increase, RR: increase
- Auscultation: decreased air movement
- Accessory muscles: severe usage
- Dyspnea: severe
- Pulsus paradoxus: >15 mmHg
- O_2 sat. <91%

Decrease inhaled albuterol to every 2 hours

- Add oral prednisone 1-2 mg/kg/dose *and*
- Continue inhaled albuterol 0.15 mg/kg/dose every 20 minutes

Admit

Observe at least 1 hour

Assess severity at 1 hour

Stable
- PEFR >70% baseline
- O_2 sat. >95% and other parameters improved

Not stable
- PEFR <70% baseline and other parameters not improved

Good response
- PEFR >70% baseline
- O_2 sat. >95% and other parameters improved

Poor response
- PEFR <40% baseline
- O_2 sat. <91% and other parameters not improved

Incomplete response
- PEFR 40-70% baseline
- O_2 sat. 91-95% and other parameters improving

Consider hospitalization

Home with patient education, medications (consider corticosteroids), and follow-up plan

Continue treatment
Consider admission if no improvement

*Therapies are often available in a physician's office. However, most acutely severe exacerbations of asthma require a complete course of therapy in an Emergency Department.
†PEFR % baseline refers to the norm for the individual, established by the clinician. This may be % predicted based on standardized norms or patient's personal best.

Figure 8–1. Asthma guidelines. (From the National Asthma Education Program. National Institutes of Health [NIH 91–3043A et al], Bethesda, MD, 1991.)

Has been cared for by her primary physician during this time and has had two to three office visits for asthmatic episodes.

Is in otherwise "good" health.

Plays daily and without limitations.

Both parents are alive and well.

Has two siblings, both well.

Family history otherwise noncontributory.

PLAN

Administer oxygen at 4 L/min via nasal cannula.

Administer *nebulized albuterol* via O_2 at 6 L/min (4.5 mg/dose) q 20 min up to maximum of 3 times in 1 hour.

Monitor vital signs, oximetry, BS, and physical signs continuously.

Monitor PEFR before and after each treatment, and use to track progress.

Provide *patient education* program information when patient and family are able to discuss this.

Clinical Notations: 9:15 AM to 9:25 AM

General Care	RC Assessments	RC Interventions	Recom- mendations
Day 1, 9:15 AM, admitted to ED Diagnosis: Asthma	Ht.: 51 in. Wt.: 60 lb. Complains of SOB. C/O exhaustion & tightness in chest. Cold symptoms noted × 2 days. Marked use of accessory muscles. HR = 148 (apical & oximetry). f = 38. BP = 110/68. Pulsus paradoxus of 20 mm Hg. BS = with distant I&E wheezing bilat. Dry cough. PEFR = 167 L/min (60% of baseline). SpO_2 = 90%. Face is flushed. Dark circles under eyes. Diaphoretic. Trembling noted. Labs pending. Allergic to pollen. npo since last noc. PMH of asthma × 2 y.	Oximetry initiated. Asthma protocol instituted.	Follow asthma guidelines. Monitor continuously. Evaluate plan after 1 h.
9:25 AM		O_2 @ 4 L/min via NC. Albuterol neb via 6 L/min O_2, q 20 min (4.5 mg/dose).	Limit treatment administration to a maximum of 3 doses over 60–90 min.

➪ **Thought Prompts**

1. Interpret the RC assessment data. Make a statement evaluating this patient's pulmonary status.

2. Which assessments will be used to guide the RC plan in this case? (Refer to Fig. 8–1.)
3. Is the current RC plan appropriate? Explain.
4. Examine each of the following and determine if the findings in this case represent good, incomplete, or poor response. Present evidence to support your conclusion.

    Auscultory findings:

    PEFR:

    Vital signs:

    Physical appearance:

5. What are the indications in this case for:
    O_2 therapy:

    Nebulized albuterol:

6. List objectives for each intervention.
7. How will each of these interventions be evaluated?
8. Are there alternatives for treatment that are not mentioned? Explain.

Clinical Notations: 9:35 AM

General Care	RC Assessments	RC Interventions	Recom- mendations
9:35 AM	Posttreatment eval: HR = 150. f = 32. Pulsus paradoxus = 10 mm Hg. Diffuse wheezing persists but is not as distant. Patient states breathing is a "little" easier. Shoulders are more relaxed in appearance with less accessory muscle use. SpO_2 = 95%. PEFR = 176 L/min (approx 65% of baseline).		Continue O_2. Maintain plan.
	Results from ABG drawn @ 9:20 AM (on 21% room air): PaO_2 = 60 $PaCO_2$ = 32 HCO_3^- = 23 pH = 7.46 SaO_2 = 90%		

➪ **Thought Prompts**

9. Have any significant improvements occurred? Explain.
10. Is the decision to maintain the plan a sound choice? Why or why not?

11. Now that the ABG results are available, make deductions concerning:

    Ventilatory status:

    Oxygenation status:

    Reliability of oximetry values:

Clinical Notations: 9:45 AM to 10:25 AM

General Care	RC Assessments	RC Interventions	Recom- mendations
9:45 AM	Albuterol indicated.	Second albuterol treatment administered, via O₂ @ 6 L/min.	
9:55 AM	Posttreatment eval: HR = 140. f = 24. Mild wheezing. PEFR = 176 L/min (approx 65% predicted). Patient states more relief. SpO₂ = 95%.		
10:15 AM		Third albuterol treatment administered as previously.	Continue plan.
10:25 AM	Posttreatment eval: HR = 126. f = 20. Mild wheezing. PEFR = 200 L/min (>75% predicted). Patient states breathing is good.		Reevaluate plan.

⇨ **Thought Prompts**

12. Describe the patient's condition at this point.
13. Was the third albuterol treatment indicated?

14. Was this treatment beneficial?
15. What recommendations would you make regarding the RC plan at this point?
16. What criteria would indicate that the patient may be discharged to home?
17. Create an RC discharge plan for this patient.
18. What educational objectives exist for use in this case?
19. How will the educational objectives be evaluated?
20. Create a list of causes associated with asthmatic episodes.
21. Describe ways in which treatment may differ according to the cause of asthma.

Summary

For a mapped summary of the major points incorporated into this case, refer to Figure 8–2. A map like this is a visual organizer for the many parts of a case like Kate Wind's.

Bibliography

AARC: Clinical practice guideline: Discharge planning. Respiratory Care 40, 1995.

AARC: Clinical practice guideline: Assessing response to bronchodilator therapy. Respiratory Care 40, 1995.

AARC: Clinical practice guideline: Pulse oximetry. Respiratory Care 36, 1991.

AARC: Clinical practice guideline: Providing patient & caregiver training. Respiratory Care 41:658–663, 1996.

Farzan, S: A Concise Handbook of Respiratory Diseases, ed 3. Appleton & Lange, Stamford, CT, 1992.

Kacmarek, R and Pierson, D: Foundations of Respiratory Care. Churchill Livingstone, New York, 1992.

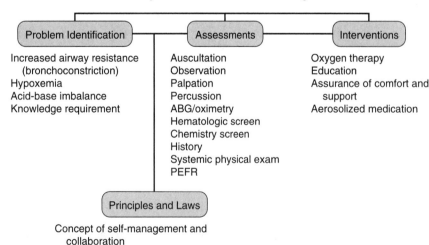

Learning Issues Related to Asthma Management

Problem Identification

Increased airway resistance (bronchoconstriction)
Hypoxemia
Acid-base imbalance
Knowledge requirement

Assessments

Auscultation
Observation
Palpation
Percussion
ABG/oximetry
Hematologic screen
Chemistry screen
History
Systemic physical exam
PEFR

Interventions

Oxygen therapy
Education
Assurance of comfort and support
Aerosolized medication

Principles and Laws

Concept of self-management and collaboration
Dalton's law of partial pressures
Critical thinking concepts for use in teaching
Poiseuille's law

Figure 8–2. A conceptual summary of learning in this case.

National Heart, Lung and Blood Institute: Managing Asthma: A Guide for Schools. National Institutes of Health. US Department of Health and Human Services, NIH Publication No. 91-2650, September 1991.

National Heart, Lung and Blood Institute: National Asthma Education Program Expert Panel Report Executive Summary: Guidelines for the Diagnosis and Management of Asthma. National Institutes of Health. US Department of Health and Human Services, NIH Publication No. 91-3042A, June 1991.

Scanlan, C, Spearman, C and Sheldon, R: Egan's Fundamentals of Respiratory Care, ed 6. Mosby, St. Louis, 1995.

Wilkins, RL and Dexter, JR: Respiratory Disease: A Case Study Approach to Patient Care, ed 2. FA Davis, Philadelphia, 1997.

PRACTICE QUESTIONS

1. Asthma may be described as either _____ or _____.
   A. Obstructive, restrictive
   B. Inferior, superior
   C. Intrinsic, extrinsic
   D. Congestive, purulent
   E. Early onset, latent onset

2. Which of the following is *not* a reliable assessment tool for monitoring the severity of an asthmatic episode?
   A. Breath sounds
   B. Diffusing capacity
   C. Peak expiratory flow rate
   D. Heart rate
   E. Color

3. The initial ABG during an acute asthmatic episode usually describes the acid-base status as:
   A. Chronic hypoventilation
   B. Severe hypoxemia
   C. Acute hypoventilation
   D. Acute hyperventilation
   E. Chronic hypoxemia

4. All of the following therapeutic agents are recommended for use during acute asthmatic episodes, except:
   A. Cromolyn sodium
   B. Albuterol
   C. Epinephrine
   D. Corticosteroids
   E. Oxygen

5. Obtain a copy of the AARC Clinical Practice Guidelines. In accordance with the CPG Selection of Aerosol Delivery Device, which of the following describes the indication for using a small-volume nebulizer in the case of Kate Wind?
   A. Need to deliver a beta-adrenergic agent
   B. Need to administer an anticholinergic agent
   C. Need to deliver an antiinflammatory agent
   D. Need to deliver a mediator-modifying agent
   E. Need to deliver a mucokinetic agent

6. Which of the following are components of clinical assessment associated with the patient's using oxygen?
   I. Vital signs
   II. Oxygen tension
   III. Oxygen saturation
   IV. Physical observation
   V. Equipment inspection at time of setup and at least daily thereafter
   A. I, II, and III
   B. I, III, and V
   C. III and V
   D. I, II, III, and IV
   E. I, II, III, IV, and V

7. What is the likely cause of the asthmatic episode in this case?
   A. Viral infection
   B. Emotional upset
   C. Inhaled irritant
   D. Cold environment
   E. Exercise

8. Which of the following are recommended for the use of a peak flow meter?
   I. The highest of two to three different measurements should be recorded.
   II. Breath in as hard and as fast as possible to perform the measurement.
   III. A standing position is preferred, if possible.
   IV. Lips should be tightly closed around the mouthpiece.
   V. Compare the value recorded to the previous best value to evaluate status.
   A. I, II, III, IV, and V
   B. I, III, and V
   C. II, III, IV, and V
   D. II, IV, and V
   E. V only

9. Asthma is a(n) _____ pulmonary disease and is associated with a decrease in _____ during acute attacks.
   A. Obstructive; expiratory flow rates
   B. Obstructive; FRC
   C. Restrictive; inspiratory flow rates
   D. Restrictive; lung volumes
   E. Obstructive and restrictive; pneumoconiosis

10. To evaluate a client's understanding of instructions in MDI use, the RCP should:
    A. Ask the family if the client is complying with the prescription.
    B. Demonstrate the procedure, and ask the client if he or she understood it.
    C. Supply written directions and have the client sign that he or she has read them.
    D. Provide a pictorial illustration of the procedure.
    E. Request that the client demonstrate the procedure.

11. An acceptable monitoring plan for home self-management of asthma would include:
    I. PEFR measurements (daily)
    II. Symptom identification and recording
    III. ABG measurements
    IV. Monitoring the environment for asthma triggers
    V. Reevaluation of the current plan at specific timed intervals
       A. I II, III, IV, and V
       B. I, II, IV, and V
       C. II and IV
       D. I, III, and V
       E. I, II, and III

ACTIVITIES

1. Using the NIH guidelines, create an outline describing an asthma education program's content. Discuss how the program may be different for differing populations, such as pediatric, geriatric, or physically challenged individuals.

2. Debate and/or discuss the use of predicted values versus actual baseline values for evaluating peak expiratory flow.

3. With a partner or group, role-play the demonstration of proper MDI administration.

9 | Dan Chan: An AIDS Patient with Pulmonary Infection

Learning Objectives

After reading the chapter and performing the activities within it, the learner will be able to:

- Identify the assessment data common to the problem of pulmonary infection secondary to AIDS.
- Create the RC plan for the case.
- Identify and discuss precautionary measures recommended for the patient and the health care provider in this case.
- Integrate the AARC's CPGs Oxygen Therapy, Bland Aerosol, Fiberoptic Bronchoscopy Assisting, and Discharge Planning into your care plan.
- Determine components essential to assisting with bronchoscopy.
- Create and sequence the RC plan.
- Consider and determine the psychosocial issues surrounding the terminally ill patient, and identify coping strategies for such a case.

Key Words and Phrases

AIDS
CD4 lymphocytes
Flexible fiberoptic bronchoscopy
HIV
Mycobacterium tuberculosis

Pentamidine
Pneumocystis carinii
Sputum induction
Trimethoprim/sulfamethoxazole

INTRODUCTION

This brief case follows the course of events undertaken during the admission of a 43-year-old man with *HIV* infection and *AIDS*. Remember, some details are omitted to enhance brevity and/or to facilitate problem solving.

Mr. Chan is admitted to the infectious disease department of a hospital and is in need of RC services for secretion mobilization, sputum induction, and oxygenation improvement. Use the clinical notations tables for gathering data in this case.

Clinical Notations: 7:10 AM

Consider items such as laboratory data to be normal if not mentioned.

General Care	RC Assessments	RC Interventions	Recommendations
Day 1, admission 7:10 AM	Patient is admitted for assessment and treatment of exacerbation of increasing dyspnea and malaise. Diagnosed with AIDS for 2 y.		
IV access initiated	Has had one hospitalization since diagnosis. Has been well otherwise. Route of HIV transmission is suspected to have been a short course of experimental IV drug use while in college— 8 y prior to diagnosis. Complains of continuous fatigue. Cachectic appearance. Complains of SOB. Uses accessory muscles for breathing. RR = 18. HR = 96. BP = 122/83. Is pale in color. Dark circles under eyes. Orthopneic, leaning forward; cannot lie flat. Lymph nodes are palpable submandibularly. Temp = 101°F. Ht. = 67 in. Wt. = 122 lb. Dry cough; states "never" produces sputum. Crackles heard bilaterally on auscultation, with decreased aeration and limited chest excursion. Percussion note is dull over RLL. CXR reveals miliary nodular pattern and an RLL consolidation. ABG on 0.21: $PaO_2 = 60$ $SaO_2 = 90\%$ $PaCO_2 = 35$ $pH = 7.45$ $HCO_3^- = 23$ $BE = 2$	Begin O_2 via nasal cannula @ 3 L/min. Initiate hypertonic saline via USN for *sputum induction.*	

ABG = arterial blood gas, AIDS = acquired immunodeficiency syndrome, BE = base excess, CXR = chest x-ray, HIV = human immunodeficiency virus, RLL = right lower lobe, USN = ultrasonic nebulizer.

⇨ Thought Prompts

1. Which of the assessments are typically associated with the diagnosis of AIDS?
2. What are the indications for the RC interventions?

   Oxygen via nasal cannula:

   Hypertonic saline aerosol:

3. Is the CXR indicative of any specific problem?
4. How should the interventions be evaluated? (What is the expected outcome?)
5. How is the oxygen administration determined?
6. What laboratory data are of essential importance in this case?
7. What precautions are required for:

   The RCP to practice:

   The protection of the patient:

8. Create the RC plan up to this time.

   Indications:

   Objectives:

   Interventions:

   Expected outcomes:

Clinical Notations: Afternoon

General Care	RC Assessments	RC Interventions	Recommendations
Day 1, afternoon	Lack of response to sputum induction. Continues to have dry cough. Patient states he is very depressed and senses that he is dying. He states he is frightened and feels confused. $SpO_2 = 96\%$.		
Bronchoscopy ordered		Equipment for bronchoscopy assembled and checked. Patient prepared. On standby for procedure.	

⇨ Thought Prompts

9. What is the indication for the bronchoscopy?
10. What is the objective for the procedure?
11. Discuss the role of the RCP in assisting with bronchoscopy.
12. Create a checklist for assembling and checking bronchoscopic equipment.
13. What adverse responses must the RCP monitor during the procedure?
14. Provide contingency plans (interventions) for each negative event that might occur.
15. Would you respond to Mr. Chan's emotional state? If so, examine your potential response from several perspectives (your own, Mr. Chan's, an observer's), and decide if it is optimal. If not, explain why.

Clinical Notations: Late Afternoon to Evening

General Care	RC Assessments	RC Interventions	Recommendations
Day 1, late afternoon IV valium	*Flexible fiberoptic bronchoscopy* completed; patient is resting. Occasional coughing noted. Patient having bronchospasm @ this time. Wheezing noted. Parameters monitored during procedure: SpO_2 = 93–95% $PetCO_2$ = 30–40 mm Hg BP = 120/85–126/86 HR = 90–100 (sinus rhythm) RR = 14–22 Samples obtained, labeled, and sent to laboratory for examination.	NRB @ 12 L/min during tx. Bronchoscopy assisting.	Provide increased O_2 delivery.
CD4 lymphocytes = 155/mm³		Return to NC @ 3 L/min. Albuterol MDI treatment.	Monitor oxygenation/ ventilation status.

Day 1: Evening meds: *trimethoprim/sulfamethoxazole*, hydrocortisone

⇨ Thought Prompts

16. Describe the patient's response to the intervention of bronchoscopy.
17. Is there an indication for any other intervention at this time? If so, what is indicated?
18. What is your recommendation at this time?
19. How would you continue to monitor Mr. Chan?
20. Hypothesize about the likely findings of this procedure. What are some likely pulmonary infections that Mr. Chan is at risk for?
21. Interpret the CD4 results.
22. What are the actions of each of the medications listed? (What problem is being treated?)
23. Was there an indication for the albuterol intervention? If so, what was it?

Clinical Notations: Discharge

Mr. Chan responds to RC and pharmacological interventions over the next week, and after 10 days a team meeting is called. Team members include the RCP, physician, nurse, and social worker. The objective is to create the discharge plan for Mr. Chan. He will be discharged to his home with medication, self-care, and a compressed-air-powered nebulizer for treatment of persistent asthmalike symptoms.

⇨ Thought Prompts

24. What is the role of each team member in this case?

25. Do you think that some roles may overlap? How and why?
26. Who are the other key team members that are not listed but will play significant roles in the outpatient care of Dan Chan?
27. What will be the objectives and expected outcomes for Mr. Chan's discharge plan?
28. Sometimes AIDS patients with CD4 levels <200 cells/mm are placed on a regimen of aerosolized *pentamidine* for prophylaxis. What specific equipment must be employed and what precautions must be included in such a therapeutic plan?
29. In what ways can the RCP prepare for work with terminally ill patients?

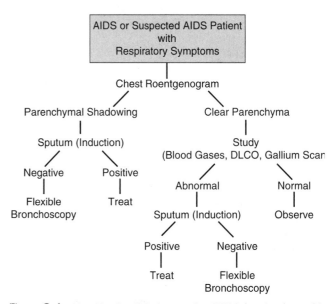

Figure 9–1. Algorithm for clinical approach to HIV-infected patients with respiratory symptoms. (From Farzan, S: A Concise Handbook of Respiratory Diseases, ed 3. Appleton & Lange, Stamford, CT, 1992, with permission.)

Examine Figure 9–2 for a conceptual summary of major points in this case.

Bibliography

AARC: Clinical practice guideline: Fiberoptic bronchoscopy assisting. Respiratory Care 38:1173–1178, 1993.

AARC: Clinical practice guideline: Bland aerosol administration. Respiratory Care 38:1196–1199, 1993.

AARC: Clinical practice guideline: Discharge planning. Respiratory Care 40, 1995.

AARC: Clinical practice guideline: Oxygen therapy. Respiratory Care 38:119, 1993.

Burton, G, Hodgkin, J and Ward, J: Respiratory Care: A Guide to Clinical Practice. JB Lippincott, Philadelphia, 1991.

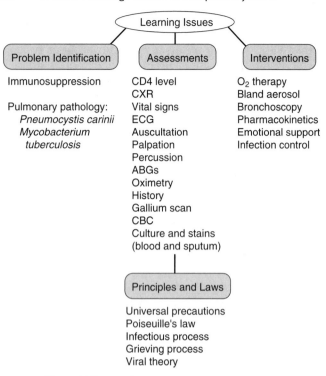

Figure 9–2. Learning issues in the case of Dan Chan.

Farzan, S: A Concise Handbook of Respiratory Diseases, ed 3. Appleton & Lange, Stamford, CT, 1992.

Luce, J: HIV, AIDS and the respiratory care practitioner. Respiratory Care 38:189–196, 1993.

Medin, D and Ognibene, F: Pulmonary disease in AIDS: Implications for respiratory care practitioners. Respiratory Care 40:833–854, 1995.

Kacmarek, R and Pierson, D: Foundations of Respiratory Care. Churchill Livingstone, New York, 1992.

Scanlan, C, Spearman, C and Sheldon, R: Egan's Fundamentals of Respiratory Care, ed 6. Mosby, St. Louis, 1995.

PRACTICE QUESTIONS

1. The infecting agent in AIDS is:
   A. Human papillomavirus
   B. *Pneumocystis carinii*
   C. Human immunodeficiency virus
   D. *Mycobacterium tuberculosis*
   E. Streptococcal bacteria

2. A critical cell count in determining prophylactic treatment as well as monitoring disease progression in AIDS is:
   A. PTT
   B. CD4
   C. RBC
   D. LDLC
   E. HPB screen

3. Pentamidine aerosolization is found helpful in preventing:

   A. *Pneumocystis* infection
   B. Tuberculin infection
   C. HIV infection
   D. A decrease in CD4 levels
   E. Global immunosuppression

4. All of the following are routinely used in the treatment of pulmonary infection in AIDS patients except:
   A. Trimethoprim/sulfamethoxazole
   B. Glucocorticoids
   C. Aerosolized pentamidine
   D. Atropine sulfate
   E. Isoniazid

5. The key practice in preventing cross-contamination in the health care setting is:
   A. Practicing good handwashing
   B. Implementing reverse precautions
   C. Using barrier devices
   D. Practicing universal precautions
   E. Ensuring proper ventilation in patient rooms

6. Which of the following is an appropriate therapeutic goal for pentamidine aerosol therapy?
   A. Maintain alveolar ventilation with $PaCO_2 < 50$ mm Hg.
   B. Induce sputum production for analysis.
   C. Maintain clear CXR.
   D. Promote bronchial hygiene.

7. Which of the following are indications for flexible fiberoptic bronchoscopy?
   I. Obtaining of sputum samples
   II. The need to measure transmural pulmonary pressures
   III. Foreign body aspiration
   IV. Assessment of the airway
   V. An aid in intubation
      A. I, II, III, IV, and V
      B. I, III, and V
      C. I, III, IV, and V
      D. I and IV
      E. II, III, and IV

8. Responsibilities involved in bronchoscopy assisting include:
   I. Setup of the scope
   II. Cleaning of the instruments
   III. Specimen retrieval and preparation for laboratory studies
   IV. Delivery of aerosolized drugs
   V. Evaluating the patient response
      A. I, II, III, IV, and V
      B. II and IV
      C. I, III, and V
      D. II, III, and V
      E. I, II, III, and V

9. Elements of proper sputum induction include:
   I. Use of hypertonic saline aerosol
   II. Ultrasonic nebulization
   III. Good patient effort

IV. Bronchoalveolar lavage and aspiration
V. Oral cavity gargling (preferably with hypertonic saline) before procedure
    A. I and III
    B. I, II, III, and V
    C. I, IV, and V
    D. II and IV
    E. I, II, III, IV, and V

10. Educational components essential to health care workers involved in the care of AIDS patients include:
    I. Disease transmission issues
    II. Current therapeutic modalities knowledge
    III. Death and dying education
    IV. Pathology concepts

V. Decision-making strategies for medical interventions
    A. I, II, III, IV, and V
    B. I, II, and IV
    C. II and V
    D. I, II, and IV
    E. II and IV

ACTIVITY

1. Investigate (individually or in a group) the grieving process. Determine the many losses that some AIDS patients may endure (loss of some friends, job, housing, security, etc.), and role-play strategies for lending support to an AIDS patient.

10 | Tom Apner: A 50-Year-Old Man with Sleep Apnea Syndrome

Learning Objectives

After reading the chapter and performing the activities within it, the learner will be able to:

- Identify the characteristic presentation of sleep apnea syndromes.
- Infer strategies for conducting diagnostic testing and performing therapeutic interventions.
- Analyze case data.
- Incorporate the polysomnography and patient and caregiver training CPGs into the case management plan.
- Make recommendations regarding the plan of care for the patient.
- Evaluate and regulate the treatment plans.
- Derive comparison and contrast assessments regarding cases presenting with similar symptoms and signs.
- Describe the process for training a patient in the use of nasal continuous positive airway pressure (CPAP) in the home.

Key Words and Phrases

Central sleep apnea
Electroencephalogram (EEG)
Electromyogram (EMG)
Electro-oculogram (EOG)
Mouth-nasal flow
Obstructive sleep apnea
    syndrome (OSAS)

Patient training
Peripheral edema
Polysomnography
Quality assurance in
    polysomnography
Quality improvement
Sleep apnea

INTRODUCTION

The following case presentation represents the progression of a simulated patient suffering from *sleep apnea* syndrome. Note that some case details are omitted to facilitate problem solving and brevity. Be sure to use a variety of resources as you work through the case.

Mr. Apner is a 55-year-old man presenting to his primary physician with a chief complaint of constant "tiredness" during the day. He states that he has been unusually agitated and tired for "quite some time"—maybe over the past year. Recently he has had difficulty staying awake at work, where he manages his own printing business, and this has prompted the office visit. He is experiencing headaches each morning. When interviewed, Mr. Apner notes that his wife complains of his loud and continuous snoring. She has been using a spare bedroom for the past several months to sleep, but she still complains of the noise.

On physical exam:

Mr. Apner is obese and pale.
Wt. = 278 lb.
Ht. = 70 in.
Temp = 98.7°F.
BP = 155/98.
RR = 17.
HR = 124.
ECG reveals sinus tachycardia with occasional PVCs.
A prominent P_2 heart sound is noted.
Percussion notes are resonant bilaterally.
BS reveal occasional crackles, scattered.
Peripheral edema noted in dependent regions.

The PMH includes chronic bronchitis with frequent upper respiratory infections. He has had one hospital admission for these problems, which occurred approximately 1 year ago.

The physician has requested laboratory studies and *polysomnography* (Fig. 10–1).

⇨ **Thought Prompts**

1. Identify the assessments that support the diagnosis of sleep apnea syndrome.
2. Are there different types of sleep apnea? If so, what are they, and how do they differ from one another?
3. What cardiac condition is implied by the assessments of peripheral edema, hypertension, and prominent P waves?
4. Describe polysomnography. What information is yielded from such a study, and how is it used?
5. Assume that you are the polysomnographic technologist. What instructions would you give to Mr. Apner, prior to the test?
6. What test findings determine the presence of sleep apnea? How is it defined?

Clinical Notations: Day 1 to Day 5

General Care	RC Assessments	RC Interventions	Recommendations
Day 1, physician's office visit	Wt. = 278 lb. Ht. = 70 in. Temp = 98.7°F. BP = 155/98. RR = 124. HR = 124 (sinus tach with PVCs). Normal chest exam. Peripheral edema. Jugular venous distention is noted. Hgb = 24 g/100 ml.	Schedule for polysomnography.	Provide written and verbal instructions.
Day 2, lab data	ABGs: PaO_2 = 60. $PaCO_2$ = 51. pH = 7.34. HCO_3^- = 25 mmol/L. WBC = 9600. CXR: Negative.	Instructions sent by fax to Mr. Apner with appointment reminder. Confirmation requested. Notation to contact patient the day before study. Also mailed map and directions.	Make follow-up call to confirm appointment, evaluate patient understanding of instructions, and reinforce key points.
Day 4		Follow-up call made. Key information clarified. Final reminders issued.	
Day 5	Temp = 98.6°F. HR = 130. BP = 160/100. RR = 18. Clear BS. No significant physical changes noted from preliminary assessment.	Preparation for study performed. Consent form discussed and signed.	Perform continuous assessment. Document entire study and submit to physician.

⇨ **Thought Prompts**

7. Analyze the laboratory data. What significant findings are present, and what do they imply?

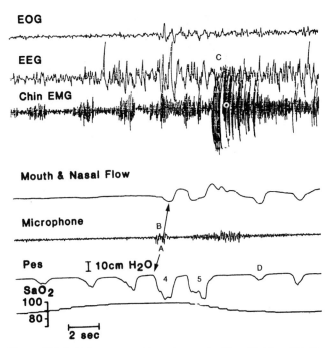

Figure 10–1. Polysomnographic tracing results. (From Fletcher, EC: Abnormalities of Respiration during Sleep. Grune & Stratton, Orlando, FL, 1986, p. 31, with permission.)

8. Discuss potential problems that should be anticipated and deterred in the study and treatment of this patient.
9. Identify essential *quality assurance* tasks that must be performed on the equipment prior to the study. How can quality be maintained and improved on a regular basis?
10. What is your interpretation of the polysomnographic tracing?
11. Is further study required? What would it entail?
12. Discuss the available treatment options for Mr. Apner.
13. What RC modality is often indicated in such cases?
14. How is the treatment plan determined?

Therapeutic modality recommended:

Settings desired:

Treatment objectives:

Evaluation of effectiveness determined by:

15. Describe instructions for a patient using nasal continuous positive airway pressure (CPAP) in the home.
16. Describe a process for choosing an appropriately fitting CPAP mask, and explain the process of maintaining the fit. (Imagine that you need to explain this to Tom Apner.)

17. Refer to the *patient and caregiver training* CPG, Section 7.2, *health care provider* (HCP) limitations, and perform self-analysis. Describe the limitations that apply to you, and suggest ways to improve the limitations. Also list those items that are not personal limitations for you.
18. What other physical problems may present with findings similar to the problem in this case?
19. Discuss long-term strategies for treating Mr. Apner's condition.
20. Analyze the tracing in Figure 10–2, performed on Mr. Apner in a follow-up examination. Create the RC plan based on your interpretation. Explain your results.
21. What occurrences would warrant a change in the RC plan?
22. How should the RC plan be evaluated?

Refer to Figures 10–3 and 10–4, a sleep apnea treatment algorithm. Notice that treatment is indicated on the basis of patient symptoms and responses. Key symptoms and signs include the number of apneas per night, cardiac status, physical condition (weight), and those physical symptoms and signs related to treatment response. Also take note that the patient condition is clustered into categories of routine (not urgent) and urgent need. In this algorithm, analysis of symptoms and general condition is used to map out the path for possible treatment of sleep apnea.

⇨ **Thought Prompts**

23. Using the treatment algorithm in Figures 10–3 and 10–4, complete the chart below:

Classification of Severity	Number of Apneic Episodes	Associated Problems	Treatment Options
Routine (not urgent):			
Urgent:			

Refer to Figure 10–5 for an overview of the learning issues in this case.

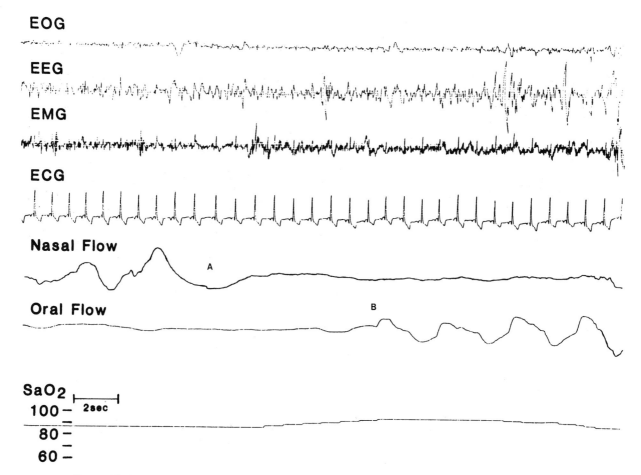

Figure 10–2. Polysomnographic tracing number 2. (From Fletcher, EC: Abnormalities of Respiration during Sleep. Grune & Stratton, Orlando, FL, 1986, p. 30, with permission.)

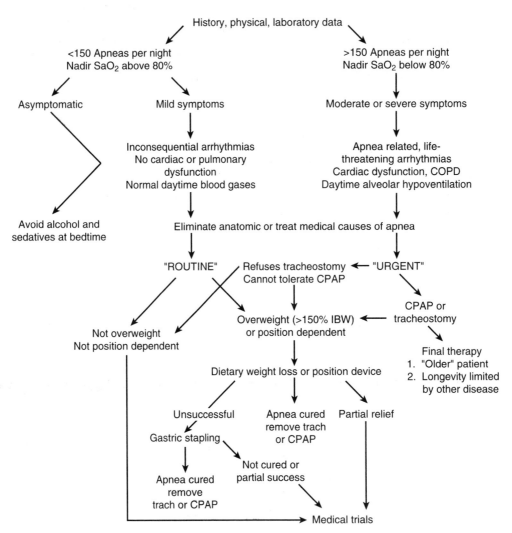

Figure 10–3. Treatment algorithm for sleep apnea. (From Fletcher, EC: Abnormalities of Respiration during Sleep. Grune & Stratton, Orlando, FL, 1986, pp. 143, 145, with permission.)

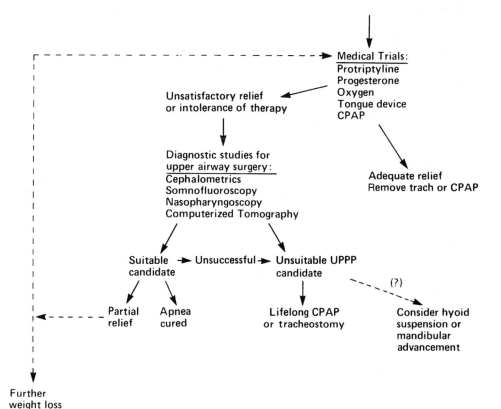

Figure 10-4. Treatment algorithm for sleep apnea (continued). (From Fletcher, EC: Abnormalities of Respiration during Sleep. Grune & Stratton, Orlando, FL, 1986, p. 147, with permission.)

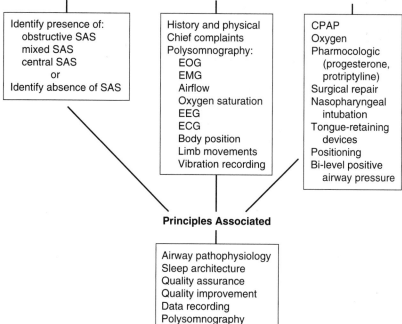

Figure 10-5. Summary of the learning issues in the case of Tom Apner.

Bibliography

AARC: Clinical practice guideline: Polysomnography. Respiratory Care 40:1336–1342, 1995.

AARC: Clinical practice guideline: Providing patient & caregiver training. Respiratory Care 41:658–663, 1996.

DesJardins, T: Clinical Manifestations of Respiratory Disease, ed 3. Mosby-Year Book, St. Louis, 1995.

Farzan, S: A Concise Handbook of Respiratory Disease, ed 3. Appleton-Lange, Stamford, CT, 1992.

Fletcher, E: Abnormalities of Respiration During Sleep. Grune & Stratton, Orlando, FL, 1986, pp. 31, 143, 145, 147.

Kacmarek, R and Pierson, D: Foundations of Respiratory Care. Churchill Livingstone, New York, 1992.

Scanlan, C, Spearman, C and Sheldon, R: Egan's Fundamentals of Respiratory Care, ed 6. Mosby, St. Louis, 1995.

Wilkins, RL and Dexter, JR: Respiratory Disease: A Case Study Approach to Patient Care, ed 2. FA Davis, Philadelphia, 1997.

PRACTICE QUESTIONS

1. Which of the following is true regarding the polysomnographic variables affected by obstructive apnea?
   A. Oxygen desaturation is the earliest of the monitored variables to reveal apnea.
   B. Oxygen desaturation occurs several seconds after other variables are displayed.
   C. EMG signals cease to be recorded during obstructive apneic periods.
   D. ECG changes associated with sleep apnea always include ventricular ectopy.
   E. Snoring is never recorded as part of a sleep study.

2. Which of the following are routinely associated with OSAS?
   I. Obesity
   II. Cor pulmonale
   III. Hypotension
   IV. Excessive daytime sleepiness
   V. Abnormal heart rhythms
   A. I, II, III, IV, and V
   B. I, III, and V
   C. I, II, IV, and V
   D. II, III, and IV

3. Which of the following are true of OSAS but *not* central sleep apnea?
   I. Absence of muscular movements are noted on EMG during apneic period.
   II. Cessation of airflow is noted during apneic period.
   III. Oxygen desaturation occurs after the onset of the apneic period.

IV. Presence of muscular ventilatory efforts during apneic period are noted on EMG.
   V. EEG and EOG tracings are used to identify stages of sleep.
   A. I, II, III, IV, and V
   B. II, III, IV, and V
   C. II and IV
   D. IV only
   E. IV and V

4. After physical assessment of a patient presenting for sleep study, you note jugular venous distention, significant hypertension, and a history of COPD. You also find that the patient is polycythemic. What problem is illustrated by this data?
   A. Myocardial infarction
   B. Pickwickian syndrome
   C. Obstructive sleep apnea
   D. Cor pulmonale
   E. Sick sinus syndrome

5. During polysomnography of a person who has been sleeping for 4 hours, the EEG tracing abruptly flattens. All other parameters remain unchanged. The technician should:
   A. Call for immediate resuscitation.
   B. Check the patient for unresponsiveness.
   C. Carefully reattach the electrode.
   D. Call the physician to perform neurological workup.
   E. Stop the study immediately and recalibrate all equipment.

6. Precautions necessary during polysomnography include:
   I. Adhesives containing collodion should not be used to attach electrodes near the eye.
   II. Calibration, maintenance, and operational verification of equipment must be performed and documented routinely.
   III. All bed rails must possess padded surfaces.
   IV. Supplemental oxygen should not be used during the study.
   V. Skin areas of electrode placement should be assessed before and after the study.
   A. I, II, and III
   B. I, II, and V
   C. II, III, and V
   D. I, III, and IV
   E. I, II, III, and IV

7. Indications for the institution of continuous positive airway pressure include all of the following except:
   A. As an adjunct in bronchial hygiene
   B. For treatment of obstructive sleep apnea
   C. To increase FRC
   D. As a method of delivering ventilation
   E. To treat apnea of prematurity

8. Acceptable objectives for CPAP intervention in the treatment of obstructive sleep apnea are:
   I. To reduce the number of sleep apnea episodes

   II. To minimize daytime somnolence as reported by patient

  III. To decrease oxygen desaturation during sleep

  IV. To minimize or prevent cardiac dysrhythmias during sleep

   V. To significantly decrease the incidence of symptoms including headache, agitation, and loud snoring

    A. I, II, III, IV, and V

    B. I, II, and III

    C. II and IV

    D. I, II, and IV

    E. I, II, III, and V

9. Alternate treatments for sleep apnea include:

    I. Weight reduction

   II. Tracheostomy

  III. Pharmacological intervention

  IV. Tongue retaining devices

   V. Sleep positioning

    A. I, II, III, IV, and IV

    B. II and III

    C. I, II, and III

    D. I, III, and IV

    E. I, III, and V

10. Indicators of polysomnographic test quality may include all of the following except:

    A. Verification of accurate calibration of devices

    B. Wide variance among technician scoring reports

    C. Routine maintenance documentation and schedule

    D. Standardization of patient preparation instructions

    E. Use of a standard policy detailing monitors and scoring

ACTIVITIES

1. Interview a local provider of respiratory home care services. Find out how services such as CPAP are ordered, delivered, and monitored for patients in the home. Discuss quality assurance and improvement measures that are standard practices within the organization.

2. Use the chart format below to compare and contrast OSAS to central sleep apnea. Graph (by hand or other tool) the wave associated with each condition. (Do not overemphasize the accuracy of your drawing, but emphasize the differences in the two graphs.)

OSAS	Central Sleep Apnea
1. Respiratory effort (abdominal, chest wall, or EMG)	
2. Airflow (nasal or oral)	
3. Oxygen saturation	

11 | Sue Hoffer: A 30-Year-Old Woman with Guillain-Barré Syndrome—A Polyneuritis

Learning Objectives

After reading the chapter and performing the activities within it, the learner will be able to:

- Recognize the clinical manifestations attributed to Guillain-Barré syndrome.
- Make evaluative judgments regarding this patient's condition and the therapeutic regimen.
- Recognize positive and negative responses to therapies.
- Determine the elements of the RC plan.
- Make recommendations about the RC plan.
- Incorporate the following clinical practice guidelines (CPGs) into the case: Oximetry, Directed Cough, Postural Drainage, Intermittent Positive Pressure Breathing, and Use of Positive Airway Pressure Adjuncts to Bronchial Hygiene Therapy.

Key Words and Phrases

Bronchial hygiene
Directed cough
Electrodiagnostics
Guillain-Barré syndrome
IPPB
Maximum inspiratory pressure (MIP)

Oximetry
Polyneuropathy
Positive airway pressure adjuncts
Tidal volume (V_t)
Vital capacity (VC)

INTRODUCTION

The following case investigates the hospital stay of a 30-year-old woman suffering from *Guillain-Barré syndrome*. Remember, parts of the record are omitted to facilitate brevity and problem solving.

RESPIRATORY CARE ADMISSION NOTE

Subjective

This 30-year-old woman reports recent history of upper respiratory infection spanning the last several days, during which she began to experience "weakness and numbness" in legs.

Objective

She presents as a healthy-looking, mildly obese woman in no respiratory distress. Is admitted and diagnosed with polyneuropathy after cerebrospinal analysis and electrodiagnostics.

Assessments on Admission

HR = 110.
RR = 16.
BP = 135/90.
Temp = 39°C.
BS are clear bilaterally.
Chest percussion is resonant over lungs.
No unusual marks are visualized.
Cough is strong and clear.
Wt. = 90 kg.

Ht. = 63 in.

CXR is negative.

Is alert and oriented.

Swallows without difficulty.

SpO_2 = 97%.

Pulmonary Mechanics:

V_t = 540 mL

FVC = 1.17 L

MIP = −53 cm H_2O

$\dot{V}_E$ = 8.1 L/min

ABG on .21 FIO_2

PaO_2 = 94 mm Hg

$PaCO_2$ = 39

pH = 7.37

HCO_3^- = 23 mEq/dL

CBC is pending.

Social History

Negative for smoking or alcohol

Walks for exercise occasionally

States being a "chocoholic"

Is married with three children (all healthy)

States has good support from home and friends

Converses in a lively and pleasant manner

Past Medical History

Three pregnancies, producing live births

Surgery for benign breast lump in 1984

No known allergies

No significant illness—only hospitalizations related to the aforementioned

Is followed yearly by primary physician

Physician-Approved Plan

Will monitor via pulmonary mechanics q 4 hr analyzing trends in data

Will perform ABGs prn

Will perform cardiopulmonary assessment q 4 hr

Evaluate plan q 24 hr

⇨ Thought Prompts

1. Given the initial assessment data, what is your judgment of this patient's condition? (Generally good, fair, or poor?) Explain.
2. Are the pulmonary "mechanics" adequate for this patient, or do they reveal a problem?
3. State a rationale for each of the interventions listed in the written plan.
4. What responses would indicate that higher levels of intervention are required?
5. Create a more extensive RC plan for this patient. Include indications, objectives, interventions, and expected outcomes.
6. Notice that several different terms are used to describe the diagnosis. Can you explain these distinctions?

Clinical Notations: 1:00 PM to 8:00 AM

Note that data not recorded may be considered normal or insignificant.

Time	General Care	RC Assessments	RC Interventions
Day 1, 1:00 PM	Diagnosis: Guillain-Barré syndrome. Admitted to general care ward.	HR = 110 RR = 16 BP = 135/90 Temp = 39°C BS = clear Normal percussion Neg CXR Clear, strong cough Wt.: 90 kg Ht.: 63 in. SpO_2 = 97% WBC = 19,000/mm³	Pulmonary mechanics: V_t = 540 mL VC = 1.17 L MIP = −53 cm H_2O $\dot{V}_E$ = 8.6 L/min ABGs: PaO_2 = 94 $PaCO_2$ = 39 pH = 7.37 HCO_3^- = 23
3:45 PM	Patient notes facial tingling. Vital signs (VS) stable. IV initiated with D5W.	SpO_2 = 98%	Mechanics: V_t = 530 mL RR = 16 VC = 1.18 L MIP = −50 cm H_2O
8:00 PM	Appears drowsy.	HR = 130 SpO_2 = 96%	Mechanics: RR = 18 V_t = 530 mL VC = 1.19 L MIP = −50 cm H_2O
12:00 AM RCP busy in the emergency department—[scheduling delay].			
2:00 AM	Difficult to arouse.	HR = 135 SpO_2 = 93% ABGs: On 0.21 RA: PaO_2 = 84 $PaCO_2$ = 45 pH = 7.35 HCO_3^- = 23	Mechanics: RR = 12 V_t = 420 mL VC = 950 mL MIP = −35 cm H_2O Increase frequency of monitoring to q 2 h
2:20 AM	Transferred to ICU.		Telephoned physician; updated and agreed on monitoring
4:15 AM	Patient asks to be allowed to sleep.	SpO_2 = 94% BS reveal ↓ aeration in lower lobes	Mechanics: RR = 12 V_t = 430 mL VC = 950 L MIP = −38 cm H_2O Explained the importance of monitoring program
6:10 AM		Cough mildly congested BS coarse over bases SpO_2 = 94%	Begin CPT with percussion and vibration q 4 h. Mechanics: RR = 14 V_t = 360 mL VC = 930 mL MIP = −36 cm H_2O
7:20 AM	Patient receives plasmapheresis.	CXR: Blunting of costophrenic angles bilat SpO_2 = 94%	

8:00 AM	$SpO_2 = 93\%$ $PaO_2 = 80$ $PaCO_2 = 44$ pH = 7.35 HR = 145 BP = 147/95	Initiate IPPB with NaCl q 2 h (using compressed air) Spontaneous mechanics: RR = 15 $V_t = 430$ mL VC = 920 mL MIP = −35 cm H_2O IPPB given with exhaled V_t @ 900 mL Cycling pressure: 20 cm H_2O Percussion and vibration also given No complaints or signs of distress noted

Bilat = bilaterally, CPT = chest physiotherapy, MIP = maximum inspiratory pressure, SpO_2 = oximetry value.

⇨ Thought Prompts

7. Evaluate the patient's condition at this point in the case.
8. What reasons exist for increasing the frequency of monitoring?
9. Determine the indications for IPPB and chest physiotherapy (CPT).
10. What are the objectives for the IPPB and CPT interventions?
11. Describe potential positive and negative responses to IPPB in this case.
12. When will these treatments be discontinued?
13. Make two separate judgments regarding the course of this polyneuropathy, one viewing a progressive trend and the other focusing on regression.
14. Is it possible that the "lateness" of the RCP at 2:00 AM had an impact on the patient's problem? Explain.
15. Consider that the RCP was performing ICU rounds at 12:00 am and then was summoned to the ER to assist in an emergency intubation. Determine possible solutions to the dilemma of needing to be in two places at one time. Make your suggestion for two separate conditions: (1) for the RCP working in a large facility with five other RCPs on the same shift and (2) for the RCP working alone in a small community hospital.

Clinical Notations: 10:00 AM to 2:10 PM

Time	General Notations	RC Assessments	RC Interventions
10:00 AM		SpO2 = 92%. HR = 140. BP = 140/93. BS course at bases. Cough is congested, producing small amounts of yellow sputum. Patient complains of difficulty swallowing.	IPPB with NaCl (@20 cm H_2O) exhaled $V_t = 900$ mL. Spontaneous mechanics: $V_t = 400$ mL VC = 1000 mL RR = 15 MIP = −36 cm H_2O

12:00 Noon		Congestion is increased, and patient expresses difficulty in coughing. $SpO_2 = 93\%$.	Directed coughing emphasized and practiced. IPPB with NaCl and 20 cm H_2O CPT with percussion and vibrations performed, including postural drainage. Patient dyspneic with "head down." Side-lying position used. Mechanics: $V_t = 420$ mL VC = 990 mL MIP = −35 cm H_2O RR = 18 Make modifications in therapy.
1:15 PM		$SpO_2 = 93\%$. HR = 135. *Directed cough produced large amount of light yellow sputum (~15 mL volume).*	IPPB exhaled $V_t = 900$ mL. Cycling pressure = 25 cm H_2O.
2:10 PM	Ambulates with RN	$SpO_2 = 93\%$. HR = 130. BS reveal coarse notes over bases, but improved aeration	IPPB given (same settings). Mechanics: RR = 14 $V_t = 450$ mL VC = 1020 mL MIP = −35 cm H_2O

Ms. Hoffer continues with q 1 h IPPB treatments until 6:00 PM, when the frequency is changed back to q 2 h. Her vital signs have improved with HR now being 120 bpm. Sputum production has decreased over the course of time, and there are only traces or streaks of light yellow color. The cough is consistently stronger, and no complaints of dyspnea have been made.

6:00 PM	Swallowing continues to be problematic	$SpO_2 = 94\%$ HR = 120	IPPB (same) Mechanics: RR = 14 $V_t = 450$ mL VC = 1045 mL MIP = −37 cm H_2O

⇨ Thought Prompts

16. Is it possible that the paralysis is reversing according to the assessments at 6:00 PM? Explain.
17. Were the changes in IPPB settings made at 1:15 appropriate? Why or why not?
18. What hazards are associated with IPPB use?
19. How would a decrease in venous return be assessed in this case?
20. What is directed coughing and how is it performed/taught?
21. Could positive expiratory pressure (PEP) therapy have been used in this case?
22. Create a map projecting a positive course for this case. Include expected outcomes.
23. Create the RC plan for the case at this juncture.

Bibliography

AARC: Clinical practice guideline: Directed cough. Respiratory care 38:495, 1993.

AARC: Clinical practice guideline: Pulse oximetry. Respiratory Care 36: 1991.

AARC: Clinical practice guideline: Intermittent positive pressure breathing. Respiratory Care 38:1189, 1993.

AARC: Clinical practice guideline: Postural drainage therapy. Respiratory Care 36:1418, 1991.

AARC: Clinical practice guideline: Use of positive airway pressure adjuncts to bronchial hygiene therapy. Respiratory Care 38:516, 1993.

DesJardins, T: Clinical Manifestations and Assessment of Respiratory Disease, ed 3. Mosby-Year Book, St. Louis, 1995.

Farzan, S: A Concise Handbook of Respiratory Disease, ed 3. Appleton & Lange, Stamford, CT, 1992.

Kacmarek, R and Pierson, D: Foundations of Respiratory Care. Churchill Livingstone, New York, 1992.

Scanlan, C, Spearman, C and Sheldon, R: Egan's Fundamentals of Respiratory Care, ed 6. Mosby, St. Louis, 1995.

Wilkins, RL and Dexter, JR: Respiratory Disease: A Case Study Approach to Patient Care, ed 2. FA Davis, Philadelphia, 1997.

PRACTICE QUESTIONS

1. Which of the following terms describes the condition examined in this case?
   A. Polyneuritis
   B. Guillain-Barré syndrome
   C. Polyneuropathy
   D. Acute polyradiculitis
   E. All of the above

2. Diagnosis of Guillain-Barré syndrome is supported by:
   A. High protein concentration in the cerebrospinal fluid
   B. Occurrence during winter
   C. Decreased expiratory flows
   D. Nonreversing paralysis
   E. Reticular granular markings on CXR

3. Relative contraindications to directed coughing include all of the following except:
   A. Inability to control possible transmission of infection from the patients suspected or known to have pathogens transmittable by droplet nuclei
   B. Elevated intracranial pressure or intracranial aneurysm
   C. Hemidiaphragmatic paralysis
   D. Reduced coronary artery perfusion, such as in myocardial infarction
   E. Acute head, neck, or spine injury

4. Indications for postural drainage include:
   I. Evidence of difficulty mobilizing secretions
   II. Increased white blood cell count (WBC)
   III. Presence of atelectasis
   IV. Presence of foreign body in the airway
   V. Inability to cough

   A. I and II
   B. II and IV
   C. I, II, and III
   D. I, III, and IV
   E. I, II, III, IV, and V

5. Which of the following are true regarding IPPB?
   I. It is not recommended for the intubated patient.
   II. It may cause pulmonary barotrauma.
   III. It should produce a V_t greater than the spontaneous one.
   IV. It is the method of choice for aerosol medication delivery.
   V. It is contraindicated when evidence of tracheoesophageal fistula is present.

   A. I, II, and III
   B. I, III, and V
   C. II, IV, and V
   D. II, III, and V
   E. I, II, III, IV, and V

6. Indications for PEP therapy include:
   I. The need to reduce air trapping in obstructive disease
   II. The need to mobilize secretions
   III. The need to reverse atelectasis
   IV. The presence of increased work of breathing
   V. The presence of hemodynamic instability

   A. I, II, and III
   B. I, III, and V
   C. II, IV, and V
   D. I, II, IV, and V
   E. I, II, III, IV, and V

7. Which of the following pulmonary data signify an intact, well-functioning pulmonary system?
   I. Spontaneous V_t = 7 mL/kg
   II. Spontaneous VC = 15 mL/kg
   III. MIP = −15 cm H_2O
   IV. RR = 35
   V. Spontaneous VC = 5 mL/kg

   A. I, III, and V
   B. II and IV
   C. I and II
   D. I, II, and IV
   E. I, II, III, and IV

8. Appointments or treatments with patients that are missed due to some unavoidable circumstance should be:
   A. Documented, signed, and placed in the patient record
   B. Disregarded because of the unavoidability issue
   C. Added on the existing schedule so as to ensure quantity
   D. Reported to the human services department for documentation in the employee record
   E. Discussed with the patient to resolve any conflict

ACTIVITIES

1. Refer to Figure 11–1 and make two statements describing: (a) An individual with very mild disease progression and (b) an individual with very severe disease progression. Include the problems that would be present prior to and during hospitalization, the assessments that would provide evidence for the mild to severe classification, and the interventions that might be used in each instance.

2. Research other disease states that may be present in similar fashion to Guillian-Barré. Describe at least two examples of similar problems and differentiate them from Guillain-Barré. (Name the problems. Explain the comparisons and contrasts. Discuss the interventions and outcomes.) Make a graphic representation of your results with, for example, a chart or concept map.

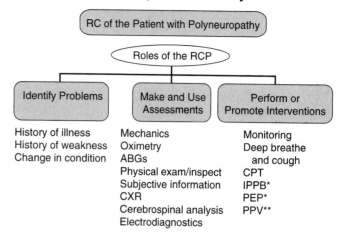

*For advancing disease.
** For severe cases.

Figure 11–1. Learning issues in the case of Sue Hoffer.

12 | Pat Garcia: A Pediatric Patient with Laryngotracheobronchitis— A Croup Syndrome

Learning Objectives

After reading the chapter and performing the activities within it, the learner will be able to:

- Recognize assessment data associated with the problem of laryngotracheobronchitis (LTB).
- Identify indicators of airway compromise.
- Recognize the indications and interventions common to LTB.
- Create outcome objectives for the case.
- Integrate into the case the CPGs for transport of the patient on mechanical ventilation (MV), management of airway emergencies, and bland aerosol administration.
- Differentiate among several upper airway problems and compare and contrast treatment regimens.

Key Words and Phrases

Continuous positive airway pressure (CPAP)
Croup syndrome
Epiglottitis
Etiology
Laryngotracheobronchitis (LTB)

Mist tent therapy
Racemic epinephrine
Stridor
Upper respiratory infection (URI)
Volume-cycled ventilation

INTRODUCTION

The following brief clinical case follows the emergency room and hospital admission of a 2-year-old child admitted for moderately severe *croup syndrome*. Some parts of the record are omitted to facilitate brevity or to prompt problem solving. Medication dosages are recorded when pertinent to the flow of the case.

EMERGENCY ROOM NOTES

Physician

A 2-year-old, 12-kg boy, admitted with barking cough, inspiratory and expiratory stridor, intercostal and suprasternal retractions, and history of upper respiratory infection (URI). Patient is crying hoarsely.

Mother states "breathing has gotten worse this evening."
Upon physical exam, patient is a well-nourished, dyspneic child, who responds appropriately to commands, has intact reflexes, and has normal heart sounds.
A-P neck x-ray exhibits marked narrowing of the subglottic region. Lateral film reveals normal epiglottis.
Hematology results are pending. RR = 32.
Temp is 38°C. Patient is negative for cyanosis and has an oxygen saturation of 92% recorded by oximeter.
Apical pulse is 140 bpm in sinus rhythm. BP = 105/70.
RC has been called for evaluation and treatment of this patient with apparent laryngotracheobronchitis (LTB).
Rule out diagnosis: Epiglottitis.

Respiratory Care Practitioner

Pulmonary assessment of this patient, as well as the history presented, supports the LTB diagnosis.

With physician consent, the RC assess and treat protocol is implemented.

Patient is found to be in urgent need.

Appears exhausted and quiet.

0.5 mL *racemic epinephrine* in 2.5 mL of normal saline via small-volume nebulizer is started. HR = 142–147 throughout treatment.

RR = 30–32.

Oxygen at 6 L/min is used to power nebulizer.

Mild improvement is noted after treatment, as assessed by decreased accessory muscle use. SpO$_2$ = 94%.

BS remain unchanged.

30% oxygen via cool *mist tent* is assembled, and patient is placed in tent. Parents are encouraged to hold patient's hand through zipper ports. Oxygen flow is adjusted to maintain 30% under these conditions.

Will reassess in 10 min, after intravenous access is achieved.

Respiratory Care Practitioner

5 min after IV placement, during which the child became quite anxious, the patient reveals further deterioration with SpO$_2$ decreasing to 90%, and cyanosis becomes apparent on lips and nail beds.

O$_2$ is increased to 60% via aerosol face mask held on child by mother. IV is in place.

ABGs performed:

(60% for 5 min)   PaO$_2$ = 63
PaCO$_2$ = 57
pH = 7.30
HCO$_3^-$ = 23
SaO$_2$ = 90%

RR = 15.

HR = 148.

BP = 85/56.

Pulse is thready to palpate.

Retractions: severe.

Nasal flaring noted.

Patient is semiconscious.

Physician

Pediatric anesthesiology resident is called to assist.

Intubation setup is ordered.

RCP concurs.

(See clinical notations for remaining case details.)

⇨ Thought Prompts

1. Which assessments made in the emergency room are specific indicators for the diagnosis of croup?
2. Record a therapeutic objective for the use of the racemic epinephrine treatment. Include the expected outcome.

3. Why is epiglottitis mentioned in this case?
4. What assessments indicate urgent need?
5. An assess and treat protocol is used in this case. Create a flow diagram summarizing this protocol.
6. Consider the use of mist tents, and create a safety checklist for their use.
7. Obtain a copy of the AARC Clinical Practice Guidelines. Using the CPG on bland aerosol administration, analyze the relationship among indications for aerosol administration (like use of a mist tent), assessment of their need, and assessment of the outcome of the intervention.
8. What evidence supports the intervention of intubation?
9. Supply the missing information in Figure 12–1.

Clinical Notations: 9:30 PM to 10:14 PM

Information not noted may be presumed normal.

Time	Physician Inputs	RC Assessments	RC Interventions	Objectives
Day 1, 9:30 PM		Patient enters ER. Intercostal retractions.		Assess.
9:40 PM	Phys exam. STAT labs. RC consult. ECG continuous. Continuous pulse oximetry.	Barking cough. I&E stridor @ rest. RR = 30. HR = 137. BP = 105/71. SpO$_2$ = 92%.	SVN: Racemic epi. (0.5 in 2.5 ml NaCl) 30% oxygen via cool mist tent	Vasoconstrict to airway edema. Maintain oxygenation. Ensure ventilation.
9:45 PM	Establish IV access.	Reactions improve after treatment with epi. IV inserted. Child cries hoarsely.		

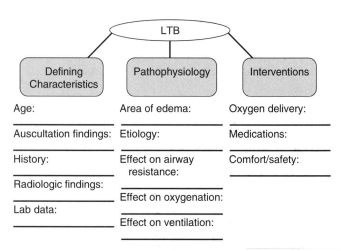

Figure 12–1. Concept map of laryngotracheobronchitis (LTB).

9:55 PM		Intercostal and suprasternal retractions noted. SpO_2 ↓ to 90%. Cyanosis appears (lips and nails).	ABGs per protocol	Assess oxygenation and ventilation.
10:03 PM	Remove tent to facilitate access to child. FIO_2.	$PaO_2 = 63$. $PaCO_2 = 57$. pH = 7.30. $SaO_2 = 90\%$. $HCO_3^- = 23$.		
10:10 PM	Call pedi anesthesia fellow STAT.	RR = 15. HR = 148. BP = 110/70. Nasal flaring. Consciousness decreasing.	60% O_2 via LVN	Improve O_2 status.
10:14 PM	Diazepam (5 mg IV). Intubate airway. Institute PPV. Intensive monitoring of cardiopulm status. CXR.	Difficult to ventilate with hand resuscitator. #4.0 oral cuffless endo tube inserted with small leak @ 30 cm H_2O PIP. *Volume-cycled vent:* SIMV RR = 10 Spont RR = 15 $V_t = 180$ mL (corrected) Spont $V_t = 60$ mL $FIO_2 = 0.50$ $V_{peak} = 18$ L/min PIP = 40 cm H_2O PEEP = 5 cm H_2O Hct: 40% Hgb: 15 g/dL Na: 140 mEq/L K: 5.0 mEq/L Ca: 10mEq/L Glucose: 60 mg/dL Creatinine: 1.1 mg/dL BUN: 6 mg/dL	Bag-mask ventilation. Intubation supplies gathered. Airway secured. PPV initiated. Perform routine airway care.	Ensure ventilation. Assist with intubation. Maintain $PaCO_2$ between 35 and 45 mm Hg. Maintain $PaO_2 > 70$. Prevent airway obstruction and/or secretion retention.

BUN = blood urea nitrogen, Ca = calcium, endo = endotracheal, epi = epinephrine, ER = emergency room, Hct = hematocrit, Hgb = hemoglobin, I&E = inspiratory and expiratory, K = potassium, LVN = large-volume nebulizer, Na = sodium, pedi = pediatric, phys = physical, PIP = peak inspiratory pressure, PPV = positive pressure ventilation, SIMV = synchronized intermittent mandatory ventilation, SpO_2 = oximetry reading, SVN = small-volume nebulizer.

⇨ **Thought Prompt**

10. Using the case data, create the RC plan for Pat Garcia at this point in the case. (Be sure to plan comprehensively, incorporating both short-term and longer-term objectives.)

Indications assessed:

Interventions:

Therapeutic objectives:

Evaluations to be performed (How will you judge the success of the plan?):

Expected outcomes:

Clinical Notations: 10:40 PM to 11:04 PM

Time	Physician Inputs	RC Assessments	RC Interventions	Objectives
10:40 PM	Maintain RC plan. Dexamethasone (12 mg IV).	Patient resting quietly. Color is improved— no cyanosis noted. $SpO_2 = 99\%$. HR = 105. Expiratory coarse wheezing. CXR reveals proper tube placement. $PaO_2 = 200$. $PaCO_2 = 40$. pH = 7.37. $HCO_3^- = 23$. $SaO_2 = 100\%$.	↓FIO_2 to 40%.	Wean O_2.
10:55 PM	Transfer to pediatric ICU (PICU).	Transport checklist completed. Color and VS stable during transport.	Transport ventilator with 50% FIO_2 used for transport.	Facilitate safe transport.
11:04 PM	PICU admission protocol.	Patient admitted to PICU.	PPV @ initial settings reinstituted as per plan and $FIO_2 = 0.40$.	

⇨ **Thought Prompts**

11. Is the decrease in FIO_2 to 0.40 indicated at 10:40 PM? Explain.
12. Notice that a transport checklist is used for transport of this intubated patient. Create such a checklist. Be concise, but include the essential points of interest.

Clinical Notations: 11:45 PM

Time	Physician Inputs	RC Assessments	RC Interventions	Objectives
11:45 PM	Stat call to pedi anesthesia and RC. Laryngoscopy/ reintubate. Diazepam (6 mg IV). Morphine (0.12 mg IV).	Severe retractions. I&E stridor. Spont $V_t = 0$. Mech $V_t = 20$ mL. Spont RR = 45. Mech RR = 0. PIP = 5 cm H_2O. HR = 170. BP = 105/67. Oral secretions markedly increased; drooling noted. Endo tube is seen to be kinked in oropharynx. Increased airway edema. 3.5 oral airway inserted—difficult intubation. Bloody secretions suctioned during procedure. No leak @ PIP of 30 cm H_2O.	Assess. Tube removed. Bag-and-mask ventilation instituted. Reinstitute PPV @ intial settings. Racemic epi (same dosage) given via inline nebulizer.	Evaluate patient condition and source of problem. Ensure oxygenation and ventilation. ↓ Airway edema. Follow original RC plan.

⇨ **Thought Prompts**

13. Was the decision to remove the tube from the child's mouth a sound choice? Why or why not?
14. Describe conditions that may have allowed the accidental extubation to occur.
15. Explain the rationale for using a #3.5 oral endo tube in this instance.
16. What is the significance of "no leak" occurring with this airway in place?

Final Clinical Notation: 5:30 AM to 6:00 PM

This child rests throughout the night and awakens at 5:30 AM. He is alert and oriented. Careful monitoring, control of sedation, and airway care are carried on throughout the day. Pat Garcia is successfully weaned from PPV and placed on *CPAP* of 5 cm H_2O and 21% FIO_2 by 6:00 PM that evening. ABGs are within normal limits, and hemodynamics are stable.

⇨ **Thought Prompts**

17. How long is this patient likely to remain intubated? Explain your answer.

18. What assessments will be used to evaluate Pat Garcia's readiness to extubate successfully?

19. Create a postextubation RC plan for this child.

20. Describe at least two upper airway conditions that may appear similar to LTB.

21. Determine the most critical differences between the care of patients you listed in response to the preceding question and the care of Pat Garcia.

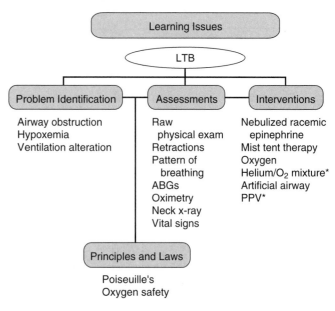

* Indicates interventions used in severe cases.

Figure 12–2. Learning issues related to LTB.

Refer to Figure 12–2 for an overview of the key concepts involved in a case such as Pat Garcia's.

Bibliography

AARC: Clinical practice guideline: Bland aerosol administration. Respiratory Care 38:1196, 1993.

AARC: Clinical practice guideline: Transport of the mechanically ventilated patient. Respiratory Care 38:1169, 1993.

AARC: Clinical practice guideline: Management of airway emergencies. Respiratory Care 40, 1995.

Barnhart, SL and Czervinske, MP: Perinatal and Pediatric Respiratory Care. WB Saunders, Philadelphia, 1995.

Kacmarek, R and Pierson, D: Foundations of Respiratory Care. Churchill Livingstone, New York, 1992.

Kurth, CD and Goodwin, SR: Obstructive airway diseases in infants & children. In: Koff, PB, Eitzman, D and Neu, J: Neonatal & Pediatric Respiratory Care. CV Mosby, St. Louis, 1988, p. 93.

McPherson, S: Respiratory Therapy Equipment. Mosby, St. Louis, 1990.

Scanlan, C, Spearman, C and Sheldon R: Egan's Fundamentals of Respiratory Care, ed 6. Mosby, St. Louis, 1995.

Thompson, JE, Farrell, E and McManus, M: Neonatal and pediatric airway emergencies. Respiratory Care 37:582, 1992.

Whaley, L and Wong, D: Nursing Care of Infants & Children. Mosby, St. Louis, 1991, p. 1440.

Whitaker, K: Comprehensive Perinatal & Pediatric Respiratory Care. Delmar, Albany, NY, 1992, p. 452.

Wilkins, RL and Dexter, JR: Respiratory Disease: A Case Study Approach to Patient Care, ed 2. FA Davis, Philadelphia, 1997.

PRACTICE QUESTIONS

1. Laryngotracheobronchitis (LTB) is usually _____ in nature.
   A. Fungal
   B. Bacterial
   C. Viral
   D. Severe
   E. Protozoal

2. The usual prodrome for LTB consists of:
   I. Upper respiratory infection (URI)
   II. Low-grade fever
   III. Gastric upset
   IV. A trunk-sparing rash
   V. Swelling at the joints
      A. I, II, III, IV, and V
      B. I, III, and V
      C. II, IV, and V
      D. I and II
      E. II and V

3. The drug of choice for inpatient treatment of LTB is:
   A. Racemic epinephrine
   B. Verapamil
   C. Tylenol
   D. Isoetharine
   E. Atropine

4. All of the following are appropriate objectives for the routine RC of LTB except:
   A. Ensure patency with artificial airway.
   B. Decrease airway edema.
   C. Maintain airway.
   D. Ensure or improve oxygenation.
   E. Maintain PaCO$_2$ between 35 and 45 mm Hg.

5. Which of the following is *not* an indicated intervention for the treatment of severe LTB:
   A. Gentamicin
   B. Racemic epinephrine
   C. Oxygen
   D. Aerosol therapy via mist tent
   E. IV access for fluid delivery

6. LTB would be considered severe when:
   I. Spontaneous tidal volume is less than 10 mL/kg of ideal body weight.
   II. PaCO$_2$ increases with a corresponding drop in pH.
   III. Inspiratory stridor is present.
   IV. Oxygen saturation <90 percent.
   V. PaO$_2$ <90.
      A. I, II, III, IV, and V
      B. I, III, and V
      C. II, IV, and V
      D. II, III, and IV
      E. I, II, and III

7. Appropriate outcome expectancies related to mist tent therapy include all of the following except:
   A. Decrease in stridor
   B. Increase in tidal volume
   C. Improved vital signs
   D. Decreased dyspnea
   E. Improved ABGs

13 | Meg Swimm: An Adolescent Near-Drowning Victim

Learning Objectives

After reading the chapter and performing the activities within it, the learner will be able to:

- Identify the primary and secondary problems associated with near drowning.
- Interpret data generated by the case.
- Interpret the signs of hypothermia and recognize interventions to treat it.
- Determine the sequence of events involved in advanced cardiac life support (ACLS).
- Identify the essential elements involved in transporting an intubated, ventilated patient.
- Recognize the therapeutic interventions indicated in the case.
- Examine the various criteria for monitoring positive end expiratory pressure (PEEP) usage.
- Create objectives and evaluations for the interventions required.
- Create an RC plan for transfer of the patient to a skilled nursing facility.
- Integrate the following AARC CPGs into the interpretation of case data: Transport of the Mechanically Ventilated Patient, Patient Ventilator System Checks, Humidification during Mechanical Ventilation (MV), Resuscitation in Acute Care Hospitals, and Discharge Planning.

Key Words and Phrases

Advanced cardiac life
   support (ACLS)
Air transport
Capnography
Defibrillation
Estimated shunt equation
Glasgow Coma Scale

Hemodynamics
Hypothermia
Long-term ventilation
Near drowning
PEEP trial
Skilled nursing facility
Tank duration

INTRODUCTION

This brief case focuses on a 14-year-old girl who experienced a submersion accident after falling through lake ice while skating with friends. Remember, parts of the record are omitted to allow the learner to experience the information-gathering process, as well as to facilitate brevity.

PARAMEDIC REPORT

This 14-year-old girl was found unresponsive, without pulse or respiration, at the scene of her fall through ice on Lake Sawtucket. The child was rescued from the freezing water by a nearby resident who heard the child's friends scream-

ing. Cardiopulmonary resuscitation (CPR) was instituted at the scene by this local resident. It is estimated that the victim was submerged for 10 to 15 min before rescue. This unit responded to emergency medical system (EMS) activation at 4:12 PM to find the aforementioned in progress. Resuscitation, ventilating with 100% oxygen, was begun. Compressions initiated. Passive rewarming instituted. Arrived at Bridgewater Community Hospital at 4:50 PM.

EMERGENCY WARD ADMISSION NOTE, CONDENSED

14-year-old, 59-in., 51-kg girl admitted after submersion in freezing fresh water. Pulseless and without spontaneous respirations. No palpable BP. Resuscitation in progress. Core temperature is 27°C presently. *Hypothermia* rescue protocol instituted. Pupils are nonreactive and dilated. Orally suctioned for vomit and grasslike matter.

>   Intubated: #8.0 oral endo tube. 100% O_2 given via hand resuscitator.
>
>   ECG: coarse ventricular fibrillation.
>
>   *Defibrillation* with 200 Joules (J). ECG unchanged.
>
>   Defibrillation with 300 J. ECG unchanged.
>
>   Defibrillation with 360 J. ECG unchanged.

IV access established: Fluids infused through warming unit.

>   Meds: Epinephrine (0.5 mL [1:10,000]
>   q 5 min IV)
>
>   Lidocaine (75 mg) IV
>
>   Defibrillation with 360 J. Sinus bradycardia with HR = 47 bpm.
>
>   Atropine (50 mg) IV.
>
>   Patient suctioned, endotracheally, for large amount brownish fluid, with particulate matter consistent with vomit and lake debris.
>
>   PPV (positive pressure ventilation) initiated.
>
>   Proximal airway temperature at 42°C.
>
>   CXR and STAT labs pending.

5:30 PM   ABGs: PaO_2 = 52
                 $PaCO_2$ = 61
                 pH = 7.10
                 HCO_3^- = 16
                 SO_2 (oxygen saturation) = 88%
                 BE = 13 mmol/L

>   IV gentamicin initiated.
>
>   Transfer to trauma center requested; granted.
>
>   Med flight expected arrival: 10 min; transfer to Northeast Medical Center.

⇨ **Thought Prompts**

1. Create the RC plan for mechanical ventilation of this patient.

Indications:

Interventions: **Objectives:**
Settings for MV:
    V_t _____
    RR _____
    FIO_2 _____
    $\dot{V}_{peak}$ _____
    PEEP _____
Safe ranges for alarm settings:
        Pressure: High _____
                   Low _____
        Oxygen: High _____
                   Low _____

PEEP: High _____
             Low _____
             Low exhaled volume ___
             Low exhaled $\dot{V}_E$ _____
Maintain airway temperature _____

Expected outcomes:

2. Examine the resuscitation actions (*advanced cardiac life support* [*ACLS*] sequence). Were these appropriate and correctly sequenced?

3. What steps must be taken to ensure safe transport of this patient? (Create a list of needed supplies and safety procedures.)

4. Discuss the particular hazards associated with *air transport* of an intubated, mechanically ventilated patient.

5. Make assumptions regarding the maintenance of oxygenation while in air transport. Present evidence to support your assumptions. (Focus on the need to maintain a given PaO_2 while increasing in altitude.)

6. Explain why maintenance of airway temperature is critical in this case.

7. Using available resources, describe methods for rewarming a patient in cases like the one presented in this chapter.

8. What is the indication for the administration of the antibiotic preparation?

9. How can the survival of this patient, submerged for at least 10 minutes, be accounted for?

10. Record your interpretation of the ABGs.

MEDICAL FLIGHT NOTATION: RESPIRATORY CARE PRACTITIONER

Full flight checklist performed.

Patient, 14-year-old, submersion incident, secured and stabilized for helicopter flight.

Patient is comatose, rated at a score of 4 on the *Glasgow Coma Scale* (App. D).

#8 oral endotrach tube is secure. Bag-mask ventilated, using 100% oxygen while transferring from *emergency ward* (EW) to helicopter. Placed on PPV:

>   RR = 12
> V_t = 700 mL
> FIO_2 = 1.00
> $\dot{V}_{peak}$ = 50 L/min
>   PEEP = 5 cm H_2O
>   Airway temp = 42°C

VS:
>   HR = 58 bpm
>   BP = 86/45 mm Hg
>   No spontaneous ventilatory attempts
>   Rectal temp = 29°C

Interventions:

> Rewarming: heated blankets; heated, humidified inspired gases; immersion heating of IV fluids; radiant heat lamp
>
> IV fluid infusion: lactated Ringer's; gentamicin IV
>
> PPV as stated
>
> Airway maintenance
>
> Monitors:
>
>> Pulse oximetry, continuous
>>
>> ECG, continuous
>>
>> Arterial line BP, continuous
>>
>> Ventilator monitors and/or alarms: Pressure, volume, RR, F_{IO_2}, temperature. All functional and accurate at this time; full check performed

Significant assessments:

> ABGs: $PaO_2 = 71$ Labs: Electrolytes
> $PaCO_2 = 47$ CBC (pending)
> pH $= 7.28$ Hematocrit
> $HCO_3^- = 20$ Hemoglobin
> BE $= 8$ mmol/L   BUN
>   Sputum anal.
>   Creatinine
>   Urinalysis
>
> Mottled coloration.
>
> BS: Moist rales bilaterally.
>
> CXR reveals reticulogranular markings.
>
> Pupils remained fixed and dilated.

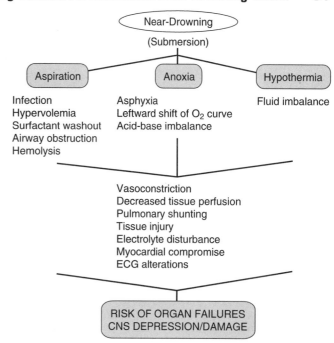

Figure 13–1. Pathogenesis of near drowning. A concept map identifying the primary and secondary problems associated with near drowning.

⇨ **Thought Prompts**

11. *Consider:* The flight from Bridgewater Community Hospital to the regional medical center takes 33 minutes. The transport ventilator requires 5 L/min (oxygen is used in this case) for maintaining functions. Will a single E cylinder be a sufficient gas supply for the trip?

12. Consider the patient's neurological status. Is it possible to attribute this condition to one problem or is it likely attributable to more than one origin? Explain. (See Fig. 13–1, the pathogenesis of *near drowning.*)

13. What is the significance of the notation "score of 4 on the Glasglow Scale"? (See App. D, Glasgow Coma Scale.)

14. Assign a Glasgow Scale rating to a patient who is *not* in as deep a level of coma as Meg Swimm. (Assign the maximum rating and take note of the variability within the scale itself.)

15. What other assessments detail the neurological status of the patient?

16. Considering that hypothermia may be a protective response, is it possible that the neurological findings are temporary, or do they reflect a permanent brain injury?

17. As the RCP, determine the primary objectives of the RC plan up to this point in the case.

For an overview of the primary and secondary problems associated with near-drowning, refer to Figure 13–1.

Clinical Notations: 4:12 PM to 6:40 PM

Values not noted may be considered "normal."

Time	Phys Exam	Labs/Imaging	RC Assessments	Interventions	Meds	Incidents
Day 1, 4:12 PM (16:12)	Unresponsive, cyanotic.		EMS activated.	RR = 12. V_t = 700 mL. F_{IO_2} = 1.00. $\dot{V}_{peak}$ = 50 L/min. PEEP = 5 cm H_2O. Airway temp = 42°C.		

Clinical Notations: 4:12 PM to 6:40 PM—*continued*

Time	Phys Exam	Labs/Imaging	RC Assessments	Interventions	Meds	Incidents
4:50 PM (16:50)	Admission to Bridgewater Community Hospital. V-fib noted by ECG. Temp (R) = 27°C. Pupils nonreactive and dilated. Vomitus and grassy substance noted in oral cavity and trachea.	STAT labs pending.	Obtunded, apneic 14-year-old girl hypothermic immersion, pulseless. Bilat BS noted, coarse crackles.	Intubated #8.0 oral ETT. Resuscitation. Defibrillation × 4. Active rewarming initiated.	IV access: Ringer's lactate infusion. Epinephrine (0.5 mL × 4). Lidocaine (75-mg bolus). Atropine (50-mg bolus). 100% oxygen. Gentamicin.	Transfer to regional facility requested and granted.
5:30 PM	Cardioversion @ 360 J. Bradycardia (HR = 58). BP = 86/45. No spontaneous RR. Temp = 29°C.	Diffuse infiltrates. On 100% O_2: PaO_2 = 52 $PaCO_2$ = 61 pH = 7.10 BE = 13 mmol/L HCO_3^- = 17	Moist rales. Central cyanosis. Stiff in posture. Mottling noted.	Witness and/or observe flight transport checklist. Ensure stability and safety prior to transport.		Transport team for flight arrives.
6:15 PM	Temp = 29°C.			In-flight monitors and equipment checked and functional.		
6:40 PM	VS and cardio-pulmonary status are stable			ECG, pulse ox, FIO_2 analyzer, MV alarms and limits—in place and functional.		Successful takeoff. No in-flight problems noted.

Bilat = bilaterally, BS = breath sounds, ETT = endotracheal tube, PPV = positive pressure ventilation, (R) = rectal temp, STAT = urgent.

Clinical Notations: 7:10 PM to 7:30 PM

Values not listed may be considered "normal."

Time	Phys Exam	Labs/Imaging	RC Assessments	Interventions	Meds	Incidents
7:10 PM	Arrival @ regional trauma center. Temp = 29.8°C. BP = 94/53. Urine output: 70 mL/h.	CXR reveals fluffy infiltrates. ABGs on arrival: PaO_2 = 68 HR = 60 $PaCO_2$ = 40 pH = 7.29 HCO_3^- = 19 SO_2 = 91% $PetCO_2$ = 28 $P_{a-et}CO_2$ = 14 HR = 60 Hgb: 15 CBC: WNL Hct: 38%	Remains unresponsive. BS coarse bilat. Chest percussion reveals dull note. Central cyanosis persists. $PetCO_2$ = 28. $P_{a-et}CO_2$ = 14. C_{st} = 14 mL/ cm H_2O. P_{plat} = 55 cm H_2O. Suctioned brownish fluid from ETT.	V_t = 700 mL (exhaled, corrected). RR = 12. FIO_2 = 1.00. PEEP = 5. MV protocol. Bronchial hygiene protocol initiated. Initiate end tidal CO_2 monitoring.	Decadron IV Gentamicin Tetanus prophylaxis	Admit to ICU.
7:30 PM		Hemodynamic data: PAP = 45/30 mm Hg PCWP = 31 mm Hg CO = 3.7 L /min $P\bar{v}O_2$ = 32 mm Hg $S\bar{v}O_2$ = 60% $C_{a-\bar{v}}O_2$ = 6.34 vol%		Patient assessment. Record review of MV system check. RR = 12. V_t = 700 mL. FIO_2 = 1.00. PEEP = 8 cm H_2O. V_{peak} = 50 L/min. Airway temp = 42°C. Alarms and limits set appropriately.		Stop active rewarming @ core temp of 34°C. A-line placed. PA-line placed.

Clinical Notations: 7:10 PM to 7:30 PM—*continued*

Time	Phys Exam	Labs/Imaging	RC Assessments	Interventions	Meds	Incidents
			$AaO_2 = 615$ mm Hg $\dot{Q}_s/\dot{Q}_t = 22\%$	and functional.		

A-line = arterial line, $C_{a-\bar{v}}O_2$ = gradient difference between arterial and venous O_2 content, CBC = complete blood count, C_{st} = static compliance, Hgb = hemoglobin, $P_{a-et}CO_2$ = the gradient between arterial and end tidal carbon dioxide, PA-line = pulmonary artery catheter, $PetCO_2$ = end tidal carbon dioxide, P_{plat} = plateau pressure, $P\bar{v}O_2$ = partial pressure of mixed venous oxygen, $\dot{Q}_s/\dot{Q}_t$ = approximate pulmonary shunt, $\bar{v}O_2$ = mixed venous, WNL = within normal limits.

⇨ Thought Prompts

18. What is the objective for performing bronchial hygiene on this patient?
19. Analyze the data presented. Determine the indications for increasing PEEP levels after arriving at the regional trauma center.
20. Describe assessments that would indicate a positive therapeutic response to the level of MV.
21. Describe assessments that would indicate a negative response to the level of MV.
22. Evaluate the pulmonary status of this patient.
23. If the patient deteriorates, what interventions may be indicated? (List more than one alternative approach and discuss the options.)
24. What problem is described by the hemodynamic data?

Clinical Notations: 7:40 PM to 10:00 PM

Time	Physical Exam	Labs/Imaging	RC Assessments	Interventions
7:40 PM	BP = 95/54 Temp = 31°C HR = 63	$PaO_2 = 62$ $PaCO_2 = 32$ pH = 7.31 $HCO_3^- = 19$ $P\bar{v}O_2 = 33$ $SO_2 = 90\%$ $AaO_2 = 618$ K = 5.9 Na = 130 Glucose = 130 Mg = 1.0 Ca = 7 mg/dL	Bilat I&E crackles PCWP = 27 CO = 4.3 $\dot{Q}_s/\dot{Q}_t = 23\%$ $C_{a-\bar{v}}O_2 = 8$ vol% $P_{a-et}CO_2 = 10$ $C_{st} = 13$ $P_{plat} = 53$ cm H_2O	PEEP = 10 $FIO_2 = 1.00$
7:55 PM	BP = 95/56 Temp = 31.5°C HR = 68	$PaO_2 = 75$ $PaCO_2 = 31$ pH = 7.47 $HCO_3^- = 20$ BE = 2 $SO_2 = 92\%$	$C_{st} = 17$ mL/cm H_2O $P_{plat} = 53$ cm H_2O $\dot{Q}_s/\dot{Q}_t = 22\%$ PAP = 36/20 PCWP = 21 $P_{a-et}CO_2 = 9$ $PetCO_2 = 22$ $P\bar{v}O_2 = 35$ $S\bar{v}O_2 = .61$ CO = 4.5 L/min Inspiratory crackles over bases only	PEEP = 12 $FIO_2 = 1.00$

| 8:05 PM | BP = 90/50 HR = 65 (sinus) Temp = 31.5°C | $\dot{Q}_s/\dot{Q}_t = 21\%$ $AaO_2 = 575$ $PaO_2 = 76$ $PaCO_2 = 37$ pH = 7.40 BE = 2 $HCO_3^- = 20$ | $C_{st} = 14$ $P_{plat} = 64$ $PetCO_2 = 26$ $P_{a-et}CO_2 = 11$ PCWP = 22 CO = 4.0 $P\bar{v}O_2 = 34$ $S\bar{v}O_2 = 60\%$ | PEEP = 14 $FIO_2 = 1.00-$ |

| 8:25 PM | BP = 96/56 HR = 68 Temp = 32°C | $\dot{Q}_s/\dot{Q}_t = 21\%$ $PaO_2 = 73$ $PaCO_2 = 37$ pH = 7.36 $HCO_3^- = 20$ | $C_{st} = 17$ $P_{a-et}CO_2 = 9$ CO = 4.3 $P\bar{v}O_2 = 35$ $S\bar{v}O_2 = 61\%$ | PEEP = 12 $FIO_2 = 0.95$ |

| 9:00 PM | BP = 100/60 HR = 70 Temp = 33°C | $\dot{Q}_s/\dot{Q}_t = 20\%$ $PaO_2 = 76$ $PaCO_2 = 37$ pH = 7.38 $HCO_3^- = 20$ | $C_{st} = 17$ $PetCO_2 = 28$ mm H_2O $P_{a-et}CO_2 = 9$ $P_{plat} = 53$ $P\bar{v}O_2 = 35$ $S\bar{v}O_2 = 61\%$ CO = 4.9 PCWP = 20 | PEEP = 12 $FIO_2 = 0.90$ |

10:00 PM   RCP notation:
FIO_2 is decreased cautiously to 0.85 by shift end (10:00 PM).

with:
$\dot{Q}_s/\dot{Q}_t = 18\%$
$PaO_2 = 76$
$PaCO_2 = 35$
pH = 7.39
$HCO_3^- = 20$
$SaO_2 = 92\%$
$P\bar{v}O_2 = 36$
$PetCO_2 = 26$
$P_{a-et}CO_2 = 9$

PEEP = 12
$V_{peak} = 50$ L/min
RR = 12
$V_t = 700$ mL
$C_{st} = 18$ mL/cm H_2O

Hemodynamics are stable at: PAP = 28/17, PCWP = 18, CO = 5 L/min.
Suctioning large amounts brownish secretions via endo tube.
Remains unresponsive. Decorticate posturing noted.
Color: Pale. Rectal temp: 34°C. BS: Crackles bilaterally over bases.
  HR: 70. BP: 100/60.
Radiant heat and immersion warming of parenteral fluids are discontinued.
Parents have visited; very distressed; express feelings of guilt and sadness.

PAP = pulmonary artery pressure, PCWP = pulmonary capillary wedge pressure.

⇨ Thought Prompts

25. Analyze the FIO_2 weaning progression. Determine the indicators for this progression. (What assessments are used to evaluate the success or failure of each change?)
26. Put yourself in the situation. You are the ICU RCP receiving report information on this patient. How will you evaluate the RC plan for MV?
27. How frequently will you recommend that the RC plan for this patient be evaluated?

Clinical Notations: Days 2 and 3

Day 2
Primary concerns for day 2 are continued weaning and maintenance of BP. The PCWP ranges from 15–19 cm H_2O. CXR is progressing toward normal with moderate general haziness remaining and a localized infiltrate reported in the right middle lobe (RML). Bronchial hygiene therapy, fluid therapy, antibiotic therapy, and maintenance of thermoregulation continue. Patient remains unresponsive to stimuli. However, brain death criteria were *not* met, as patient exhibits minimal ventilatory efforts when challenged.

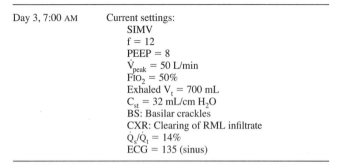

Day 3, 7:00 AM   Current settings:
                     SIMV
                     f = 12
                     PEEP = 8
                     $\dot{V}_{peak}$ = 50 L/min
                     FIO_2 = 50%
                     Exhaled V_t = 700 mL
                     C_{st} = 32 mL/cm H_2O
                     BS: Basilar crackles
                     CXR: Clearing of RML infiltrate
                     $\dot{Q}_s/\dot{Q}_t$ = 14%
                     ECG = 135 (sinus)

Clinical Notation Summary: Day 4 to Day 25

Patient's course of treatment has been a lengthy one. Patient required full MV support. Tracheostomy performed on day 18 of hospitalization. Current settings: SIMV: f = 12, V_t = 700 mL, FIO_2 = 35%, and 6 PEEP. Patient has required continuous antibiotic therapy and aggressive bronchial hygiene to manage recurrent pulmonary infections. Due to unstable ventilatory drive, this patient has required full MV support. She remains in coma but exhibits nonpurposeful movements of her limbs and takes occasional deep breaths spontaneously. Responds to painful stimuli but not to command. Requires full assistance for bodily functions.

This 14-year-old girl is to be transferred to "Willow" *skilled nursing facility* for continued care. Parents have been supportive and are assuming parts of her care. Both are professionals in the computer technology industry. They express concern regarding the transfer but are pleased that their child will be in a facility closer to their home. They also express the desire to care for their daughter at home, with assistance, as soon as possible.

⇨ Thought Prompts

28. Create the discharge plan for this child. Include objectives for treatment, interventions, method and schedule for evaluation, and any recommendations that you might have.

29. What educational objectives exist for the parents of this child?

For a summary of the learning issues involved in a case like Meg Swimm's, refer to Figure 13–2.

Bibliography

AARC: Clinical practice guideline: Transport of the mechanically ventilated patient; and Resuscitation in acute care hospitals. Respiratory Care 38:1169, 1993.

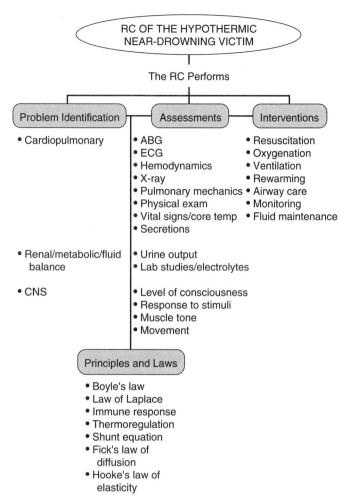

Figure 13–2. Learning issues in the case of Meg Swimm.

AARC: Clinical practice guideline: Humidification during MV; and Patient ventilator system checks. Respiratory Care 37, 1992.

AARC: Clinical practice guideline: Discharge planning for the respiratory care patient. Respiratory Care 40, 1995.

AARC: Clinical practice guideline: Providing patient and caregiver training. Respiratory Care 41, 1996.

Burton, G, Hodgkin, J and Ward, J: Respiratory Care: A Guide to Clinical Practice. JB Lippincott, Philadelphia, 1991.

DesJardins, T: Clinical Manifestations and Assessment of Respiratory Disease, ed 3. Mosby-Year Book, St. Louis, 1995.

Farzan, S: A Concise Handbook of Respiratory Diseases, ed 3. Appleton & Lange, Stamford, CT, 1992.

Kacmarek, R, Hess, D and Stoller, JK: Monitoring in Respiratory Care. Mosby, St. Louis, 1993.

Kacmarek, R and Pierson, D: Foundations of Respiratory Care. Churchill Livingstone, New York, 1992.

Scanlan, C, Spearman, C and Sheldon, R: Egan's Fundamentals of Respiratory Care, ed 6. Mosby, St. Louis, 1995.

Wilkins, RL and Dexter, JR: Respiratory Disease: A Case Study Approach to Patient Care, ed 2. FA Davis, Philadelphia, 1997.

PRACTICE QUESTIONS

Using resources relied on throughout this case, answer the following questions.

1. What is the correct sequence for treatment of ventricular fibrillation?
   I. Defibrillate @ 360 J.
   II. Perform CPR.
   III. Defibrillate @ 200 J.
   IV. Administer lidocaine.
   V. Defibrillate at 200 to 300 J.
   A. I, II, III, IV, and V
   B. II, III, V, I, and IV
   C. V, II, III, I, and IV
   D. II, IV, III, V, and I
   E. I, II, V, IV, and III

2. Obtain a copy of the AARC Clinical Practice Guidelines. According to the CPG on transport of the mechanically ventilated patient, hazards and complications associated with this procedure include the following:
   I. Equipment failure can result in inaccurate data or loss of monitoring capabilities.
   II. Movement may result in accidental extubation.
   III. Hypoventilation during manual ventilation may cause respiratory alkalosis, cardiac dysrhythmias, and hypotension.
   IV. Movement may result in accidental removal of vascular access.
   V. Loss of oxygen supply may lead to hypoxemia.
   A. I, II, III, IV, and V
   B. I, II, III, and IV
   C. II, III, IV, and V
   D. I, II, IV, and V
   E. I, III, and V

3. Which of the following events represents a factor that correlates to successful use of PEEP?
   A. Increase in blood pressure
   B. Decrease in cardiac output
   C. Decrease in arterial to end tidal gradient
   D. Increase in PCWP
   E. Decrease in urine output

4. Which of the following is required to calculate an estimated shunt?
   I. CaO_2
   II. SO_2
   III. PCWP
   IV. PaO_2
   V. FIO_2
   A. I, II, III, and IV
   B. I, III, and V
   C. I, II, IV, and V
   D. II, IV, and V
   E. II and IV

5. Which of the following medications may *not* be administered via endotracheal tube in an emergency resuscitation?

   A. Bretylium
   B. Epinephrine
   C. Lidocaine
   D. Naloxone
   E. Atropine

6. Select the information needed to compute a static compliance:
   I. Peak inspiratory pressure
   II. Corrected tidal volume
   III. Plateau pressure
   IV. PEEP
   V. Peak flow
   A. I, III, and V
   B. II and IV
   C. II, III, and IV
   D. II and III
   E. I, II, III, IV, and V

7. The hemodynamic factor most reflective of left heart function is:
   A. PAP
   B. BP
   C. PCWP
   D. RAP
   E. CVP

8. All of the following are likely causes of pulmonary edema except:
   A. Hypovolemia
   B. Near drowning
   C. Head injury
   D. Ventricular failure
   E. Pulmonary aspiration

9. The normal gradient between arterial and end tidal carbon dioxide ($P_{a-et}CO_2$) is:
   A. 18 mm Hg
   B. 4.5 mm Hg
   C. 12 mm Hg
   D. 25 mm Hg

ACTIVITY

Review the manipulation of PEEP levels in this case, and make an inference as to the data that correlate to the optimal level of PEEP. Explain your thoughts.

Time	5:30	6:15	7:10	7:30	7:40	7:55	8:05	8:25	9:00	10:00
PEEP	5	5	5	8	10	12	14	12	12	12
PaO_2	52		68		62	75	76	73	76	76
$\dot{Q}_s/\dot{Q}_t$				22	23	22	21	20	20	18
$P\bar{v}O_2$				32	33	35	34	35	35	36
$P_{a-et}CO_2$			14		10	9	11	9	9	9
BP	86/45		94/53		95/54	95/56	90/50	96/56	100/60	100/60
CO					4.3	4.5	4		4.3	5
PCWP				31	27	21	22		20	18
C_{st}			14		13	17	14	17	17	18
Temp (core)	29°C	29°C	29.8°C	31°C	31.5°C	31.5°C	32°C	33°C	34°C	
HR	58		60		63	68	65	68	70	70
FIO_2	1	1	1	1	1	1	1	0.95	0.9	0.85

14 | Mabel Cash: A 65-Year-Old Woman with Acute Myocardial Infarct

Learning Objectives

After reading the chapter and performing the activities within it, the learner will be able to:

- Identify the presenting signs and symptoms of a myocardial infarction (MI).
- Recognize and interpret assessments associated with the problem of MI.
- Determine appropriate assessment strategies for the case.
- Make professional inferences regarding the progression of the case.
- Interpret case data to form conclusions and make care planning judgments.
- Interpret electrocardiograph (ECG) tracings in the case.
- Create an RC plan for this case.
- Assess the similarities and differences of problems presenting like MI.

Key Words and Phrases

Cardiac enzymes
Cardiac history
Electrocardiograph (ECG)
Emergency medical system (EMS)
Hemodynamic data

Intraaortic balloon counterpulsation (IABC)
Mechanical ventilation (MV)
Myocardial infarction (MI)
Oxygen therapy
Streptokinase

INTRODUCTION

The following case represents the progression of a simulated patient having an acute myocardial infarction (MI). Some details are omitted to facilitate brevity and to allow problem solving. Remember to use the tables within the chapter and additional resources to follow the medical description of events. This case in particular will require research outside of the "usual" scope of reading.

Mabel Cash is a 65-year-old woman who, upon waking and walking her dog, began experiencing severe chest pain, shortness of breath, and high anxiety. Her husband activated the local emergency medical system (EMS), and Ms. Cash was transported with oxygen via nasal cannula at 2 L/min to a local hospital emergency department (ED).

RESPIRATORY CARE EMERGENCY DEPARTMENT ASSESSMENT

8:35 AM.
Patient presents with chest pain: severe.

Diaphoretic.
HR = 169.
RR = 32.
Dyspneic and orthopneic.
BP = 105/69.
SpO_2 = 80%.
ABGs pending.
ECG: ST-segment elevation, inverted T waves, and presence of Q waves in leads I, aV_L, and V_1 through V_6.
Patient complains of nausea.
Laboratory studies pending.
IV access established.

⇨ Thought Prompts

1. In view of the data presented, what immediate interventions are indicated, and why are they indicated?
2. Is the electrocardiogram (ECG) representative of a particular problem? If so, describe the condition.
3. What assessments in combination with the ECG data support your conclusion?

4. How would you plan to assess this patient further?
5. What are some associated problems to be aware of and watch for?

AVAILABLE PATIENT HISTORY

8:55 AM.

The patient is dyspneic but reports the following as answers to questions. (Husband also provides some data.)

- Patient is alert and oriented.
- Pain has been present for about 40 min.
- Is severe in nature.
- No medications were taken at home today.
- Follows daily medication regimen for known high BP.
- Has history of chronic bronchitis "from smoking."
- Has been advised by primary physician to reduce weight while adhering to a low-cholesterol diet.
- Has an 80-pack-per-year smoking history.
- States having frequent indigestion lately.
- Both parents died from "heart attacks."
- Has one sibling who has had coronary artery bypass surgery at age 59.
- Has five children.

➡ **Thought Prompt**

6. Are any additional risk factors for the patient's condition noted in the history?

Clinical Notations: 8:35 AM

General Care	RC Assessments	RC Interventions	Recom-mendations
Day 1, 8:35 AM, admitted to ED via ambulance. ED physician, RCP, and nurse assess and treat. Diagnosis: Suspected acute anterior transmural MI Ventricular irritability Central venous catheter placed. IV medications: Nitroglycerin Morphine sulfate Propranolol Lidocaine *Streptokinase*	Patient presents with chest pain: severe. Diaphoretic. HR = 169. RR = 32. Dyspneic and orthopneic. BP = 105/69. SpO_2 = 80%. ECG: ST-segment elevation, inverted T waves and presence of Q waves in leads I, aV_L, and V_1 through V_6. Frequent premature ventricular contractions (PVCs) noted. Patient complains of nausea. Laboratory studies pending.	100% O_2 initiated via nonrebreathing oxygen mask (NRB) @ 12 L/min. ABGs performed and pending. 12-lead ECG done and recorded. IV access established.	Oxygen via NRB @ 12 L/min. Improve oxygenation. Reassess as lab data is reported and according to observation of patient. Prepare for the need to intubate and mechanically ventilate the patient.

Clinical Notations: 8:55 AM to 9:05 AM

General Care	RC Assessments	RC Interventions	Recom-mendations
8:55 AM, medical record accessed. Primary physician arrives.	History: Smoker (80 pack/y). Known chronic bronchitis. Baseline ABGs do not indicate CO_2 retention. Known elevated LDLC. + for high BP and on medication for control. Family history of cardiac disease. Ht.: 62 in. Wt.: 195 lb. ABGs: PaO_2 = 53 $PaCO_2$ = 54 pH = 7.25 HCO_3^- = 21 SaO_2 = 84% FIO_2 @ 1.00 via NRB @ 12 L/min Patient losing consciousness.		Intubate and place on MV.
9:05 AM	Bilat BS noted. Few crackles scattered.	Intubation with #8 oral endo tube. Hand resuscitation initiated. Called second RCP to respond with MV and verify operation.	Request CXR. Monitor closely.

ED = emergency department, LDLC = cholesterol measure, NRB = nonrebreathing oxygen mask, + = positive for.

➡ **Thought Prompts**

7. What assessments support the diagnosis of MI?
8. Identify the indications for intubation and MV.
9. Determine appropriate ventilatory settings for the patient:

   Mode: _____

   V_t: _____

   f: _____

   FIO_2: _____

   $\dot{V}_{peak}$: _____

   PEEP: _____

   Alarm settings and limits: _____

   _____

   _____

10. Create objectives for the RC plan for this case.
11. Streptokinase, a thrombolytic agent, is used in this case. Determine its indication and action. What negative effects of thrombolytic therapy does the RCP need to be mindful of?

Clinical Notations: 9:25 AM

General Care	RC Assessments	RC Interventions	Recommendations
9:25 AM, Patient is transferred to cardiac procedure laboratory. Pulmonary artery catheter is inserted. Request for assistance in *IABC* initiation.	BP ↓ to 75/54. Patient becomes unconscious. SpO₂ reads 75%, but signal is weak. HR = 134. RR = no spontaneous efforts. Urine output = 12 mL/hr. RAP = 16 mm Hg. PAP = 35/18. PCWP = 20. CI = 1.7 L/min/m². P$\bar{v}$O₂ = 30 mm Hg.		Alert RC supervisor of need for RC coverage in ED.

CI = cardiac index, *IABC = intraaortic balloon counterpulsation*, PAP = pulmonary artery pressure, PCWP = pulmonary capillary wedge pressure, RAP = right atrial pressure.

⇨ Thought Prompts

12. What problem is indicated by the *hemodynamic data*? Note the CI.
13. Is it likely that this problem is associated with the MI?
14. Is the urine output indicative of a problem?
15. Identify the problems in the above clinical notations that may in part be attributed to or aggravated by positive pressure ventilation.
16. Describe the essential equipment and precautions that must be taken in transporting a patient with this condition.
17. What are the goals associated with use of an intraaortic balloon counterpulsation (IABC)?
18. Make inferences regarding the role of the RCP in assisting with IABC (pump) operation. What advanced-level skills are essential to the practitioner?
19. Determine positive therapeutic effects of the treatment regimen at this point in the case.

20. Determine negative effects that might occur.
21. How are good time and resource management skills exhibited by the RCP in this case so far? (See data in the clinical notations tables.)

Clinical Notations: Day 15

Mabel Cash undergoes successful IABC therapy and then requires coronary artery bypass surgery. She recovers appropriately from the events and procedures and is scheduled for discharge on day 15.

⇨ Thought Prompts

22. Describe three therapeutic goals that must have been achieved before Mabel Cash could be discharged.
23. Describe two personal risk management strategies that the RC department may assist the patient with in this case.
24. Determine appropriate outcome criteria for the outpatient care of this patient.
25. What psychological issues may need to be addressed in an MI case?

Table 14–1   NORMAL VALUES FOR CALCULATED HEMODYNAMIC DATA

Mean arterial blood pressure (MAP)	80–100 mm Hg	$\dfrac{\text{Systolic} + (2 \times \text{diastolic})}{3}$
Pulse pressure	40 mm Hg	Systolic − diastolic
Stroke volume (SV)	60–100 mL	Cardiac output (CO)/h
Cardiac index (CI)	3.5–4.5 L/min/M²	CO/BSA
Oxygen content, arterial (CaO₂)	20 vol%	%sat × Hgb × 1.34
Oxygen content, venous (C$\bar{v}$O₂)	15 vol%	%sat × Hgb × 1.34
Arteriovenous oxygen content difference (C$_{a-\bar{v}}$O₂)	5 vol%	CaO₂ − C$\bar{v}$O₂
Oxygen transport	1000 mL/min	CO × CaO₂
Oxygen consumption (VO₂)	200–300 mL/min	CO × C$_{a-\bar{v}}$O₂

Adapted from Kiess-Daily, E and Speer Scroeder, J: Techniques in Bedside Hemodynamic Monitoring, ed 5. Mosby, St. Louis, 1994.

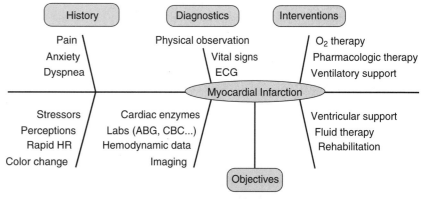

Figure 14–1. Concept map of the case elements.

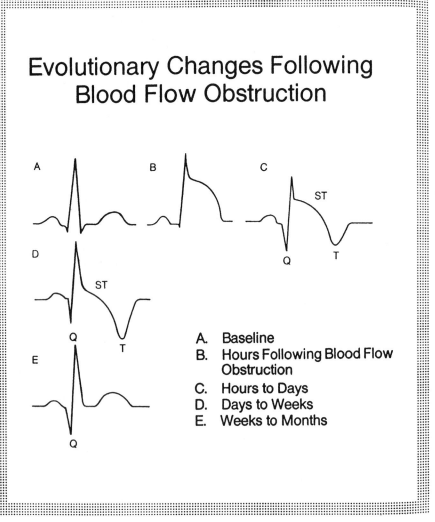

Evolutionary Changes Following Blood Flow Obstruction

A
B
C   ST
D   ST
         Q   T
E

A. Baseline
B. Hours Following Blood Flow Obstruction
C. Hours to Days
D. Days to Weeks
E. Weeks to Months

Figure 14–2. ECG changes associated with myocardial infarction. Note that the ST segment elevation occurs prior to the formation of the Q wave. During these early hours, interventions are often undertaken to reverse the process. As time passes, the Q wave forms, the ST segment is less elevated, and the T wave inverts. The final outcome varies greatly, depending on the amount of myocardial damage. (From Stein, E: Clinical Electrocardiography. Lea & Febiger, Malvern, PA, 1987, p. 140, with permission.)

Bibliography

Collins Abrams, A: Clinical Drug Therapy. Rationale for Nursing Practice, ed 2. JB Lippincott, Philadelphia, 1987.

Cummins, RO (ed): Textbook of Advanced Cardiac Life Support. American Heart Association, Dallas, 1994.

Finkelmeier, BA: Cardiothoracic Surgical Nursing. JB Lippincott, Philadelphia, 1995.

Keiss-Daily, E and Speer Scroeder, J: Techniques in Bedside Hemodynamic Monitoring, ed 5. Mosby, St. Louis, 1994.

Phillips, R and Feeney, M: The Cardiac Rhythms, ed 3. WB Saunders, Philadelphia, 1990.

Pilbeam, S: Mechanical Ventilation. Mosby, St. Louis, 1992.

Stein, E: Clinical Electrocardiography. Lea & Febiger, Philadelphia, 1987.

PRACTICE QUESTIONS

1. When a person in his or her home complains of chest pain that is not easily relieved, the appropriate action is:
   A. Call the physician immediately.
   B. Drive to the nearest hospital.
   C. Activate EMS.
   D. Administer nitroglycerin.
   E. Begin chest compressions.

2. The ECG changes associated with myocardial infarction include:
   I. ST-segment elevation
   II. Disappearance of P waves
   III. Inversion of T waves
   IV. Appearance of Q waves
   V. Appearance of wandering baseline
      A. I, II, and III
      B. I, II, III, and IV
      C. I, III, and IV
      D. II and III
      E. I, II, III, and V

3. All the following are risk factors contributing to coronary artery disease except:
   A. Female gender
   B. Obesity
   C. Smoking
   D. Elevated LDLC
   E. Sedentary lifestyle

4. Which of the following are appropriate RC objectives for oxygen therapy?
   I. Maintain $SaO_2 > 90\%$.

Table 14–2 **NORMAL HEMODYNAMIC PRESSURES**

	Unit	Normal Value	How Measured	Use
Heart rate (HR)	bpm	60–90	Watch	Early index of tachycardia and bradycardia
Blood pressure (BP) (systemic)	mm Hg	Systolic: 90–140 Diastolic: 60–90	BP cuff or arterial line	Early index of hypertension or hypotension
Central venous pressure (CVP)	mm Hg	1–6	From CVP catheter or PA 3- or 4-lm catheter	Estimates right ventricular preload; also for drug and fluid administration
Pulmonary artery pressure (PAP)	mm Hg	Systolic: 15–25 Diastolic: 5–15	From PA catheter	Measures pulmonary vascular resistance (PVR)
Pulmonary capillary wedge pressure (PCWP)	mm Hg	5–12	From PA catheter in occluded position (balloon inflated)	Estimates left ventricular filling and preload
Cardiac output (CO)	L/min	5–8	By thermodilution or dye dilution	An important determinant of hemodynamic function
Mixed venous partial pressure of oxygen ($P\tilde{v}o_2$)	mm Hg	40	From distal tip of PA catheter	Overall assessment of cardio-pulmonary function
Arterial partial pressure of oxygen (Pao_2)	mm Hg	80–100	From a systemic artery	Assesses level of arterial oxygenation

Adapted from Deshpande, VM, Pilbeam, SP and Dixon, RJ: A Comprehensive Review in Respiratory Care. Appleton & Lange, Stamford, CT, 1988, p. 358.

Table 14–3 **ENZYME ELEVATIONS AFTER MYOCARDIAL INFARCTION**

Finding	Creatine Kinase	Creatine Kinase-MB	Lactate Dehydrogenase
Rises (hours)	4–8	4–8	8–12
Peaks (hours)	12–24	12–20	72–144
Returns to normal (days)	3–4	2–3	8–14

Adapted from Lee, TH and Goldman, L: Serum enzyme assays in the diagnosis of acute myocardial infarction. Ann Intern Med 105:221, 1986.

    II. Decrease myocardial oxygen demand.
    III. Maintain oxygen transport > 1000 mL/min.
    IV. Ensure Pao_2 > 90 mm Hg.
    V. Maintain cardiac index > 3.0 L/min/m^2.
        A. I, II, III, IV, and V
        B. I, II, and III
        C. II and IV
        D. I, III, and V
        E. II, III, and IV

5. All the following assessments describe cardiogenic shock except:
    A. Cardiac output < 4.5 L/min
    B. Cardiac index < 2.0 L/min
    C. Urine output < 20 mL/h
    D. Hypotension
    E. Tachycardia

6. In the following illustration, identify the pulmonary artery (PA) tracing.

A

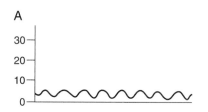

B

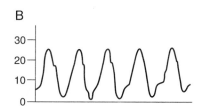

C

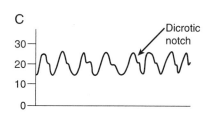

7. If you noted the following pressure tracing after balloon deflation of a pulmonary artery balloon flotation catheter, you should:
    A. Do nothing; this is normal.
    B. Flush the catheter line.
    C. Perform calibration procedures.
    D. Draw a blood sample from the distal port.
    E. Withdraw the catheter slightly until a notched tracing appears.

A

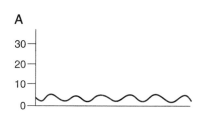

8. When a patient is on positive pressure ventilation, he or she may experience the adverse effects of:
    I. Decreased transmural heart pressures
    II. Increased urinary output
    III. Decreased renal perfusion
    IV. Hyperinflation of the lungs
    V. Gastric irritation
       A. I, III, and V
       B. II and IV
       C. I, II, III, IV, and V
       D. I, III, IV, and V
       E. I, II, and IV

9. Identify the enzymes routinely used in diagnosing and monitoring myocardial infarction:
    A. Creatine kinase; lactate dehydrogenase
    B. Diabinese; Cardizem
    C. Prostaglandin; Pulmozyme
    D. Carbonic anhydrase; cardiase
    E. Myogenase; Diabinase

10. Which of the following are not useful assessments of infection related to invasive monitoring?

    A. Increased white blood cell (WBC) count
    B. Increased platelet count
    C. Positive culture of catheter tip
    D. Positive blood culture
    E. Increase in body temperature

ACTIVITIES

1. Because this case followed the early stage of this cardiac problem, *cardiac enzyme* monitoring was not addressed in depth. Therefore, for greater understanding of the clinical monitoring of an MI patient, explain why these blood levels are repeated in a serial fashion. Examine the reason for elevations in their levels, and grasp the usefulness of this knowledge. Then create an intervention plan incorporating the assessments as monitoring tools. (What would the goal be? What would you monitor? How would you know improvement from regression?)

2. Compare this short case to one related to mitral regurgitation. Note the similarities as well as the differences. Record your findings. (A chart would serve well.)

15 | Matt Babson: A 76-Year-Old Postsurgical Patient with Chronic Obstructive Pulmonary Disease— A Pulmonary Rehabilitation Case, Subacute to Home Care

Learning Objectives

After reading the chapter and performing the activities within it, the learner will be able to:

- Create and monitor the RC plan for subacute care.
- Create and monitor the care plan for the home care of this client.
- Create the discharge plan for this client.
- Interpret and use assessment data to determine interventions and achievement of objectives.
- Make inferences regarding regulation of the RC plan.
- Integrate into the case the AARC CPGs on exercise testing of hypoxemia, oxygen therapy in the home, and spirometry.
- Recommend educational objectives and content used in pulmonary rehabilitation.
- Infer troubleshooting strategies for equipment used.
- Assemble and check home care equipment for proper function.
- Create plan for assisting with the mobility of the home care client.
- Document home care visits appropriately.

Key Words and Phrases

Activities of daily living (ADLs)
Chronic obstructive pulmonary disease (COPD)
Continuum of care
Discharge planning
Liquid oxygen
Long-term oxygen therapy (LTOT)
Mobility of the home care client
Noninvasive positive pressure ventilation (NIPPV)
Pulmonary rehabilitation
Respiratory home care
Screening documentation
Subacute care

INTRODUCTION

The following case represents the *subacute care* and *respiratory home care* of a patient with *chronic obstructive pulmonary disease (COPD)* who recently underwent abdominal surgery. Remember, some details are omitted to faciliate brevity as well as problem solving. Be sure to use a variety of resources, including the recommended readings at the end of this chapter, to assist you in following the case.

Mr. Babson is a 76-year-old retired electrician entering a subacute facility specializing in the care of persons with respiratory diagnoses. Mr. Babson is 8 weeks postoperative from emergency resection of abdominal aneurysm surgery. He sustained a diaphragmatic injury intraoperatively, as well. He has a significant history of COPD. He has a 3-year history of *long-term oxygen therapy (LTOT)*, using low-flow oxygen approximately 8 to 10 hours per day (nocturnally). Mr. Babson spent 2 weeks on MV and was weaned using pressure support. Since extubation, he has required *noninvasive positive pressure ventilation* (NIPPV) *nocturnally* and *continuous low-flow oxygen* to maintain SaO$_2$ > 85%. He has been unable to perform routine self-care functions since his surgery.

Table 15–1 contains the screening documentation gathered by the RCP from the subacute facility.

⇨ **Thought Prompts**

1. Interpret the physical assessments on Mr. Babson. Identify his primary pathological problems.
2. Classify Matt Babson's pulmonary condition using the assessment scoring system in Table 15–2. Determine if he is in poor, fair, or good condition. (Note that this is *not* a valid scoring instrument but a learning tool.)
3. Determine an appropriate short-term goal and long-term goal for Mr. Babson's subacute care.
4. Develop the RC plan for this subacute resident at this time.

Indi-cations	Objectives	Inter-ventions	Outcome evaluations

5. Determine appropriate settings for NIPPV in this case.
6. Using available rehabilitation resources, describe the essential components of a rehabilitation program that could benefit Mr. Babson.
7. Incorporate your current plan into a discharge plan for Mr. Babson. Consider the RC plan's objectives as a starting place.
8. Identify potential discharge planning team members.
9. Describe the components of a breathing retraining program.
10. This facility does not have "piped-in" oxygen and instead uses *liquid oxygen.* What are the advantages and disadvantages of such a system?
11. What would Mr. Babson use as an oxygen source to ambulate and exercise with? How would this be assembled and checked for operation? Describe an RC policy that should be implemented for the patient's ambulatory needs.

Table 15–1 **SCREENING DOCUMENTATION**

History	Activity History	Physical Exam
Ex-smoker— 90 pack/y. Quit smoking × 16 y. Diagnosed with COPD × 20 y. Has had 2 admissions in the last 4 y for COPD. Has used low-flow oxygen @ noc × 3 y. Recurrent pneumonias × 25 y. Postcholecystectomy —1987. Postappendectomy —1970. *Family:* Lives with wife of 50 y. Has 2 sons and 3 daughters. Has been "very" active with 12 grand-children—attending sporting events, playing, gardening and wood-working with them. Visits weekly. *Occupational:* Electrician for a large depart-ment store chain; retired × 9 y. Until present illness, active with local volunteer group driving truck to deliver furniture to needy families. *Recent illness:* Post–abdominal aortic aneurism (AAA) resection. PPV × 2 wk. Weaned using pressure support ventilation (PSV). Meds: Anxiolytics, antacids, inhaled corticosteroids, and benzodiazepine @ noc. Has used nocturnal NIPPV since surg to maintain PaO$_2$ > 60 with PaCO$_2$ < 70 and norm pH. Continuous oxygen (low flow) has been needed. Adrenergic MDI used 9.4 h and prn for bronchospasm.	Walked daily × 2 mi. Woodworking in own workshop daily. Maintained all self-care up until recent surgery. Active with retiree club, attending monthly luncheons. Active weekly, attending functions with grandchildren. Habits: Quit smoking, has an occasional social drink.	Moderately cyanotic, thin 76-year-old man. Ht.: 70 in. Wt.: 150 lb. Dyspneic @ rest, using accessory muscles. Has oxygen via cannula @ 2 L/min on continuously. Is alert and states being depressed with illness. BS are decreased bilaterally. RR = 16. HR = 106. Temp = 37°C. BP = 155/95. Increased anterior-posterior (AP) diameter with hyperresonant percussion note. Decreased rib expansion. CXR: Hyperaeration. PFT: Reduced FEV$_1$ (50%) Reduced DLCO (58%) RV = 120% Exercise testing: Desaturation occurs after 3 min walking and breathing room air. Hct: 45%. Hgb: 19. ABGs: PaO$_2$ = 65 PaCO$_2$ = 66 pH = 7.36 HCO$_3^-$ = 42 On O$_2$ @ 2 L/min.

Clinical Notations: First 2 Weeks

Mr. Babson progresses well over the next 2 weeks and meets the set objectives. However, one morning it is noted that Mr. Babson's nasal mask, a standard type of mask on the market, has left skin excoriation around the bridge of his nose.

Table 15-2 **SCORING SYSTEM**

Assessments	Good Condition, 1	Fair Condition, 2	Poor Condition, 3
Ability to perform activities of daily living (ADLs)	Performs all self-care	Requires some assistance	Cannot perform ADLs
Level of dyspnea	No dyspnea	Dyspnea on exertion	Continual dyspnea
Duration of required supplemental O_2 use	None or only used with exercise	<12 h/day (nocturnal)	Continuous
PFT	Mild disease	Moderate disease	Severe disease
Exercise testing	Tolerates 6 min of walking	Walks @ least 3 min without desat	Cannot perform
Other organ system problems	None	One other system with problem	>1 other system with problem

⇨ Thought Prompts

12. Identify the likely cause of Mr. Babson's skin excoriation.
13. Describe the appropriate action to correct the condition.
14. Regulate the RC plan. (Update it and implement any changes necessary.)
15. Provide an example of how this problem should be documented, and explain where this documentation should be placed.

Clinical Notations: Discharge

Matt Babson is ready for discharge to home. He will reside with his wife. His daughter who lives nearby will visit daily.

⇨ Thought Prompts

16. What criteria should be met for the discharge to occur?
17. In administering an exercise stress test, what hazards may exist?
18. Adjust the *discharge plan* to the current needs of Mr. Babson.
19. What must be included in Mr. Babson's oxygen prescription?
20. In preparation for his transition to home, describe essential factors for Mr. Babson's wife and daughter.
21. Describe the components of Mr. Babson's educational plan for home care.
22. Describe the essential tasks the RCP must perform to assist Mr. Babson with his transition to home.

23. Do any further assessments need to be gathered?
24. You would like to recommend an oxygen-conserving device to Mr. Babson. Discuss available options and describe their operation.

Clinical Notations: Arrival at Home

Mr. Babson arrives home and has his initial in-home assessment by the home care RCP.

⇨ Thought Prompts

25. What data will be collected by interview at this point?
26. What physical assessments will be required?
27. How will the environment be evaluated? What recommendations may need to be made?
28. How will the equipment be assembled and checked for proper function?
29. What recommendations should be made to Mr. Babson at this point?
30. How should Matt Babson be evaluated for his level of understanding of the plan of action and his own role in it?
31. How often should Mr. Babson be visited by his home care RCP?
32. What should take place during these visits?
33. What backup equipment and/or strategies should be on hand for Mr. Babson in case of need?
34. What is the primary role of the home care RCP? Is it intervention oriented or evaluation oriented? Explain.

Clinical Notations: 3 Months Later

After 3 months at home, with good progress, Mr. Babson requires nocturnal NIPPV and oxygen @ 2 L/min during exercise and ambulation. He has decided to visit his son in another state. A 2-h plane ride will be involved, as well as a week's stay with his son and family.

⇨ Thought Prompts

35. Recommend management strategies for this situation.
36. Describe the services that must be coordinated to ensure that Mr. Babson will have a safe and enjoyable trip.

Refer to Figure 15-1 for a summary of the concepts of this case.

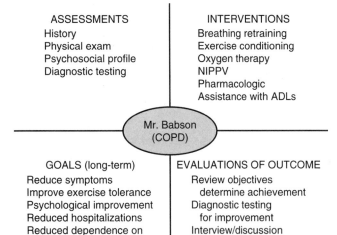

ASSESSMENTS
History
Physical exam
Psychosocial profile
Diagnostic testing

INTERVENTIONS
Breathing retraining
Exercise conditioning
Oxygen therapy
NIPPV
Pharmacologic
Assistance with ADLs

Mr. Babson
(COPD)

GOALS (long-term)
Reduce symptoms
Improve exercise tolerance
Psychological improvement
Reduced hospitalizations
Reduced dependence on
technology

EVALUATIONS OF OUTCOME
Review objectives
    determine achievement
Diagnostic testing
    for improvement
Interview/discussion
Physical examination
Continued data collection

Figure 15–1. Concepts of the case of Matt Babson.

Bibliography

AARC: Clinical practice guideline: Oxygen therapy in the home or extended care facility. Respiratory Care 37:918, 1992.

AARC: Clinical practice guideline: Exercise testing for evaluation of hypoxemia and/or desaturation. Respiratory Care 37:907, 1992.

AARC: Clinical practice guideline: Spirometry. Respiratory Care 36:1414, 1991.

AARC: Clinical practice guideline: Providing patient & caregiver training. Respiratory Care 41:658–663, 1996.

AARC: Clinical practice guideline: Long-term invasive mechanical ventilation in the home. Respiratory Care 40:1313, 1995.

Bickford, L, Hodgkin, J and McInturff, S: National pulmonary rehabilitation survey. J Cardpulm Rehabil 15:406, 1995.

Celli, B: Physical reconditioning of patients with respiratory diseases: Legs, arms and breathing retraining. Respiratory Care 39:481, 1994.

Kacmarak, R: Foundations of Respiratory Care. Churchill Livingstone, New York, 1992.

Leger, P: Noninvasive positive pressure ventilation at home. Respiratory Care 39:501, 1994.

Lucas, J, Golish, J, Sleeper, G and O'Ryan, J: Home Respiratory Care. Appleton & Lange, Stamford, CT, 1988.

May, D: Rehabilitation and Continuity of Care in Pulmonary Disease. Mosby, St. Louis, 1991.

Miller, A: Pulmonary Function Tests. Grune & Stratton, Orlando, FL, 1987.

Scanlan, C: Fundamentals of Respiratory Care, ed 6. Mosby, St. Louis, 1995.

PRACTICE QUESTIONS

1. Which of the following illustrations represents an obstructive component displayed by the flow-volume loop?

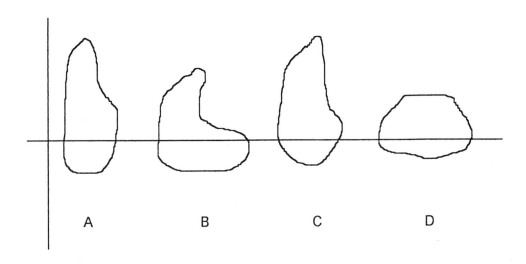

A   B   C   D

2. All of the following are devices for conserving oxygen except:
   A. Transtracheal catheter
   B. Pulse dose device
   C. Borg scale
   D. Reservoir cannula

3. Which of the following best evaluates the client's understanding of transfilling a portable oxygen (LOX) cylinder?

   A. He states that he completely understands.
   B. He is observed transfilling his portable unit.
   C. He writes out the steps and signs his name.
   D. His family tells you he is quite competent at this procedure.

4. Given the following data, make an interpretation: ABG on 0.21; $PaO_2 = 56$; $PaCO_2 = 45$; pH = 7.47; and $HCO_3^- = 33$.

   A. Mixed acidosis (metabolic and respiratory)

B. Chronic hypoxemia with metabolic acidosis
C. Respiratory failure
D. Respiratory alkalosis superimposed on chronic respiratory acidosis
E. Respiratory acidosis superimposed on respiratory alkalosis

5. Given a situation in which a noninvasive ventilation system is not delivering the prescribed inspiratory pressure, which of the following is the most likely problem?
A. A leak at the humidifier
B. A poor mask fitting
C. A leak at the nebulizer
D. An obstruction in the patient's trachea
E. A kink in the circuit

6. If a patient has a full LOX and runs oxygen at 1 L/min, how long will it take before the tank is ½ full (approximately)? The cylinder weight is 2 lb.
A. 11 hours
B. 5.5 hours
C. 600 hours
D. 12 hours
E. 1 day

7. Given the same situation, but using an E cylinder, how long will it take before it is ½ full?
A. 5 hours
B. 3 hours
C. 60 minutes
D. 10 hours
E. 600 hours

8. Which of the following signs should be reported to the physician of a home care patient?
I. Change in sputum consistency
II. Increased level of dyspnea
III. Edema of the ankles
IV. Nocturnal diaphoresis
V. Fever
A. I, II, III, IV, and V
B. I, III, and V
C. I, II, and III
D. I, II, III, and V
E. II and V

9. Current guidelines for reimbursement of home oxygen include:
A. Presence of $SaO_2 < 85\%$
B. $PaCO_2 > 50$ mm Hg
C. Documented respiratory failure
D. Presence of congestive heart failure
E. Presence of sleep apnea

10. If an RCP were to receive a rebate for the referral of a home oxygen therapy patient, the RCP would:
A. Have no conflict of interest
B. Need to document all remunerations for tax purposes
C. Need to document the rebate in the patient record
D. Be guilty of a felony

ACTIVITIES

1. Interview providers of home RC services and supplies. Investigate the reimbursement process that must occur. Describe the documentation required for such reimbursement, and explain the criteria for various services such as oxygen therapy and/or NIPPV.

2. Visit and investigate a local subacute facility offering RC services. Describe the types of RC interventions that are provided. Compare and contrast these services to those routinely offered in hospital or at home. Describe any differences.

16 | Elle Carey: An 18-Year-Old Victim of Multiple Trauma with Head, Neck, and Chest Injuries

Learning Objectives

After reading the chapter and performing the activities within it, the learner will be able to:

- Perform RC assessment in the emergency setting.
- Analyze, interpret, and evaluate patient data.
- Create and regulate the RC plan.
- Explain the rationale for interventions in the case.
- Create and adjust the discharge plan.
- Make inferences regarding the source of problems occurring in the case.
- Participate in the critical care and discharge planning team treating and supporting this patient.
- Integrate the AARC CPGs into the case: Discharge Planning, Long-Term Invasive Mechanical Ventilation in the Home, Capnography/Capnometry during MV, Defibrillation during Resuscitation, Ventilator Circuit Changes, Transport of the Mechanically Ventilated Patient, Resuscitation in Acute Care Hospitals, Endotracheal Suctioning of Mechanically Ventilated Adults, Patient-Ventilator System Checks.

Key Words and Phrases

Advanced cardiac life
    support (ACLS) drugs
Advanced cardiac life
    support (ACLS) resuscitation
Defibrillation
Electrocardiography

Glasgow Coma Scale
Hemodynamics
Intracranial pressure (ICP)
Long-term MV
Pleural drainage

INTRODUCTION

The following case represents the course of events surrounding an 18-year-old female victim of multiple trauma. Ms. Carey was struck by a motor vehicle while standing at a bus stop near her home.

Remember, some parts of the record are not presented, either for brevity or to create an opportunity for problem solving.

INITIAL RESPIRATORY CARE ADMISSION ASSESSMENT

This 18-year-old woman is admitted with multiple injuries sustained in a traffic accident that "pinned" Ms. Carey between a building and an automobile. She was conscious at the scene. Was brought to ED via ambulance. Resuscitation was initiated during transport by emergency medical technician (EMT), as indicated by cessation of spontaneous breathing. Oral airway was placed, and ventilation was noted to be evidenced by the presence of bilateral BS. Basic life support (BLS) ongoing. Massive hemoptysis noted.

Admission data:

BR = not distinguishable by sphygmomanometer.
RR = no spontaneous respirations.
HR = no palpable pulse.
Temp = 35°C
Level of consciousness: Nonresponsive.
Pupils are dilated but reactive, with R more enlarged than L and less reactive.

BS: Moist rales bilaterally with absent aeration over left chest (during bag-mask ventilation).

Physical appearance: Obvious lacerations covering face, head, chest, and limbs. Asymmetrical chest movement noted when ventilated. Left foot is angled at 90° from the midline.

Palpation: Crepitus felt over left and right chest. Oral and nasal cavitites filled with blood. Left clavicle appears displaced posteriorly.

100% oxygen via hand resuscitator; increasingly difficult to ventilate; marked increase in pressure required to deliver a breath.

Unable to intubate orally or nasally.

Laryngeal edema noted by laryngoscopy.

Bloody drainage from left ear.

⇨ Thought Prompts

1. There are two RCPs, two nurses, two resident physicians, and one ED physician in attendance. Describe the likely roles of the RCPs in this situation.

2. Prioritize this patient's current needs. (What are the most urgent interventions indicated?)

3. Analyze and interpret the electrocardiography (ECG) tracing in Figure 16–1. Integrate the other available assessments, and decide if *advanced cardiac life support (ACLS)* should be instituted.

4. If ACLS is initiated, what is the sequence of events? (Explain the algorithm that should be used.)

5. Consider that an obvious head injury is present. What associated injuries must be anticipated and managed?

6. In cases of increased *intracranial pressure (ICP)*, what MV strategy is often employed?

7. If IV access were not available, what other routes are available for administration of *ACLS drugs?*

8. Are dosages affected by administering medication via a different route?

9. What options exist for assuring airway patency?

10. Make an inference regarding the chest assessments. (What is the likely problem, and how should it be addressed?)

11. Use the *Glasgow Coma Scale* (see App. D) to assign a coma level rating to Elle Carey.

12. Identify other scoring systems that rate the severity of illness or trauma.

Clinical Notations: 4:20 PM to 4:30 PM

General Care	RC Assessments	RC Interventions	Recommendations
Day 1, 4:20 PM Resuscitation V-tach protocol. ABGs drawn.	No spontaneous RR. No pulse. BP not palpable. T = 35°C. Not responsive to stimuli. Pupils are dilated but reactive. R > L. Hemorrhaging from head and face. Bloody ear drainage. Admission for mult trauma: head, chest, ?neck, limbs, ?abdominal. Laryngeal edema noted. BS absent over L chest during hand ventilation. Crepitus palpated over upper chest and L shoulder. Rales over rest of chest.	Resuscitation with 100% O₂. *Defibrillation* per protocol. Oral and nasal intubation failure due to airway edema and deformities.	Assess and treat according to ACLS guidelines. Maintain airway with present device; prepare for alternate artificial airway insertion.
4:30 PM, type and cross-matching, CBC, electrolytes, BUN, pro-thrombin, glucose pending. IV fluids initiated via subclavian catheter. Second IV line placed. ACLS meds administered. Mannitol administered. Blood transfusion begun. Foley catheter inserted. Tracheostomy performed, size #8 mm.	Rhythm change after 360-J shock. BP = 75 systolic by doppler. 220 mL bloody urine measured Ventilations are increasingly difficult to perform.	Institute ACLS protocol for present ECG rhythm. Trach tube positioned and checked.	

ACLS = advanced cardiac life support, ECG = electrocardiograph, R > L = right pupil more dilated than left, 360 J = 360-joule shock applied.

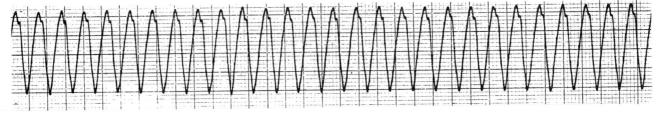

Figure 16–1. ECG tracing number 1, Elle Carey.

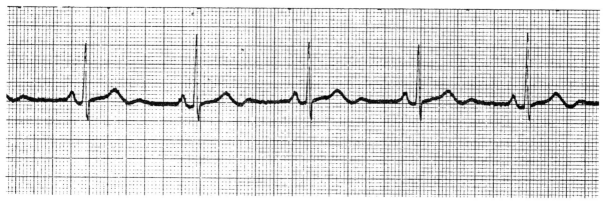

Figure 16–2. ECG tracing number 2, Elle Carey.

⇨ **Thought Prompts**

13. Describe verification procedures for checking the position and patency of an artificial airway.
14. Present evidence supporting the choice of tracheostomy in this case.
15. Why, in your opinion, is the ventilation increasingly difficult?
16. What are some likely root causes of the problem described in the preceding question?
17. Analyze and interpret the ECG tracing in Figure 16–2 and recommend treatment.

Clinical Notations: 5:15 PM

General Care	RC Assessments	RC Interventions	Recommendations
5:15 PM, dopamine administered. NG tube inserted. L chest tube inserted. IV infusion continues. Request to transport to CT scan and surgical trauma OR.	ECG change occurs. HR = 88. BP = 91/62 (with dopamine). IBW = 75 kg. Suctioning >50 mL bloody, frothy fluid from trach tube. CXR confirms L pneumothorax and L hemothorax. ABG (@ 4:27 PM): PaO$_2$ = 55	Continue ventilation. MV initiated. Chest drainage unit assembled, checked, and connected to patient.	Initiate MV. Monitor: All critical care patient parameters. Monitor: Interventions and equipment according to policy.

Physician requests bronchoscopy setup and PA-line insertion setup.
Parents arrive and visit quickly. RN accompanies them to waiting area to update and interview.

PaCO$_2$ = 71
pH = 7.20
HCO$_3^-$ = 23
50 mL bloody drainage from chest tube.
Urine output: 23 mL.
Actual wt.: 77 kg.

IBW = ideal body weight.

⇨ **Thought Prompts**

18. Analyze and interpret the ECG tracing (Fig. 16–3) recorded at 5:15 PM. Explain the correct plan of action based on the ECG tracing.
19. Describe your plan for mechanically ventilating this patient. (Include ventilator settings and outcome objectives, and describe any specific techniques that should be used.)

Objectives:	Interventions/ settings:	Expected outcomes:

20. How often should the ventilator-patient system be checked?
21. What should be assessed during these checks?

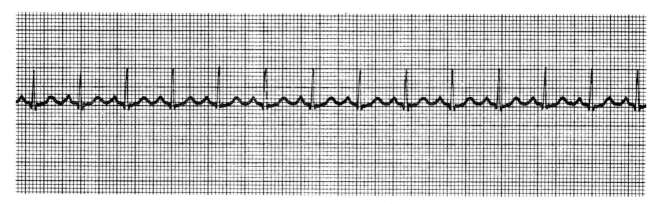

Figure 16–3. ECG tracing number 3, Elle Carey.

22. How frequently should ventilator circuits be changed?
23. What would the airway care of the patient involve?
24. Create a checklist for the assembly and operational verification of fiberoptic bronchoscopy equipment.
25. What complications of bronchoscopy are serious risk factors for this patient?
26. Describe the supplies and equipment that would need to be gathered, assembled, and checked for the insertion of a PA-line.
27. What procedures would need to be performed to check the function of the PA-line equipment?
28. What essential tasks must the RCP perform for the safe transport of this patient?
29. Complete the RC plan below:

Objectives:	Interventions (include monitors):	Expected outcomes:

1. Ensure airway patency, ventilation, and oxygenation.
2. Promote resolution of pneumothorax and reexpansion of lungs.
3. Monitor and maintain normal *hemodynamic* values.
4. Promote neurological recovery.
5. Prevent infection and promote patient safety.
30. What essential items will need to be removed for disinfection, cleaned, checked, or restocked in the emergency department?

Clinical Notations: 8:00 PM to 11:00 PM

General Care	RC Assessments	RC Interventions	Recommendations
8:00 PM, Intra-op data. Dopamine discontinued.	Ventilated with: V_t = 800 mL, RR = 19 bpm, FIO_2 = 60%, PIP = 50–55, PaO_2 = 79, $PaCO_2$ = 21, pH = 7.55, HCO_3^- = 22, BP = 120/73 mm Hg, CO = 5.8 L/min, CI = 3.4 L/min/m², SVR = 1330 dynes × sec × cm⁻⁵, PVR = 166 dynes × sec × cm⁻⁵, RAP = 10 mm Hg, PAP = 16 mm Hg, PAWP = 12 mm Hg, Urine output: 40 mL/h		

11:00 PM, IV infusing continuously. Procedures performed: craniotomy for evacuation of subdural hematoma, laminectomy, thoracotomy, and bronchoscopy. Fracture reductions: Maxillary, nasal, zygomatic, and L tibia. Line insertions: PA, arterial. ICP monitor inserted. Cervical traction applied. Furosemide administered.	Patient admitted from OR to SICU. Ht. 68 in. Wt. = 78 kg. Obtunded. Diagnostic findings: Subdural hematoma, vertebral fractures of C-5 and C-6. Laryngeal obstruction due to edema from crushing injury; pulmonary contusion; myocardial contusion. Multiple fractures: maxillary, nasal, zygomatic, tibial, ribs: # 4, 5, 6, and 7 on L and # 6 on R side. Urine output = 31 mL/h. No spontaneous RR. HR = 95 (sinus). Crackles auscultated bilat. BP = 125/75 mm Hg, PAP = 46/26 mm Hg, PAWP = 24 mm Hg, CO = 6 L/min, CI = 3.5 L/min/m², SVR = 1120 dynes × sec × cm⁻⁵, PVR = 160 dynes × sec × cm⁻⁵, ICP = 18 mm Hg	Assess patient. Verify ventilator operation and connect to patient airway. Perform system check. Verify monitor operation and connect ECG, PA-line, and A-line. Verify airway placement and patency. Check cuff.

BUN = blood, urea, nitrogen, C-5 and C-6 = cervical vertebrae, CI = cardiac index, CO = cardiac output, Ht. = height, Wt. = weight, ICP = intracranial pressure, OR = operating room, PA-line = pulmonary artery catheter, PAP = pulmonary arterial pressure, PAWP = pulmonary arterial wedge pressure, PIP = peak inspiratory pressure, PVR = pulmonary vascular resistance, RAP = right atrial pressure, SICU = surgical intensive care unit, SVR = systemic vascular resistance.

➪ Thought Prompts

31. What is indicated by the hemodynamic data?
32. What is the likely cause of the problem?
33. What is the indication for furosemide?

Clinical Notations: Patient's Transfer to ICU

General Care	RC Assessments	RC Interventions	Recommendations

As patient is transferred to the ICU bed from the transport bed, the *pleural drainage* unit is dropped to the floor and rolled upon by the transport bed. It is cracked and draining upon the floor.

➪ Thought Prompts

34. What action should the RCP take at this point to manage the pleural drainage problem?
35. How should the action be evaluated?

Clinical Notations: 12:30 AM

General Care	RC Assessments	RC Interventions	Recommendations
12:30 AM	ABGs: $PaO_2 = 70$ $PaCO_2 = 22$ pH = 7.55 $HCO_3^- = 22$ Suctioning small amounts of blood-tinged sputum from trach tube. PAP = 29/15 mm Hg. PAWP = 11 mm Hg. CO = 5.7 L/min. ECG: Sinus @ 90. BP = 126/75 mm Hg. No spontaneous RR. Remains unresponsive to stimuli. Eyes are swollen shut. ICP = 17. Urine output: 45 mL/h. Wt.: 77 kg. BS reveal few crackles; aeration improved.	Assess/perform vent check. Interpret ABGs and recommend changes. Perform airway care. Analyze hemo-dynamic data and document.	

The patient's father asks the RCP if his daughter has a good chance of recovering without brain damage. He also asks about withdrawal of MV if recovery is unlikely.

➭ Thought Prompts

36. From the perspective of the RCP in this scenario, examine the options available for discussing the issues with Elle Carey's father.
37. Evaluate the spinal injuries. Describe the likely outcome of such injuries.
38. Describe methods to prevent increases in ICP.
39. If the PA-catheter distal tip were positioned so that it was higher than the monitoring transducer, what error would occur?

Clinical Notations: 5:00 AM to Day 3

General Care	RC Assessments	RC Interventions	Recommendations
Stable assessments and checks recorded throughout shift.			
5:00 AM	FIO_2 = 40%.	MV RR decreased to 12 bpm.	
5:20 AM, chest tube removed.	ABGs drawn.		
Day 3	PAP = 24/12. PAWP = 10. CO = 5.5 L/min. Urine output = 43 mL/h clear. ICP = 15. FIO_2 = 30%. PaO_2 = 90. $PaCO_2$ = 35. pH = 7.39. HCO_3^- = 22. BP = 123/89. Pupils are reactive; patient focuses intermittently.		

➭ Thought Prompts

40. Consider the ventilator rate reduction. Is this an appropriate recommendation at this time?
41. Evaluate the progress or regression of the patient at this time.

After considerable time and medical care, Elle Carey makes some progress. Read the final clinical notation, and make recommendations according to the thought prompts.

Clinical Notations: Day 52

General Care	RC Assessments	RC Interventions	Recommendations
Day 52	Patient and family are ready for discharge to home. *Long-term MV* plan is activated. Patient uses sip and puff wheelchair with portable MV attached; reveals competency in use. Confirms knowledge of safety issues.	Final evaluation of patient and family occurs.	Provide all documentation and recom-mendations to home care RCP/agency. Determine follow-up focus areas.

➭ Thought Prompts

42. Describe the patient and family condition(s) that must exist for successful transition to home MV.
43. Identify the essential components of the long-term MV plan.
44. How might the case outcome differ if Elle Carey did not have family members willing to participate in her care? If she were intubated orally at this time? If she did not regain consciousness?

Bibliography

AARC: Clinical practice guideline: Patient-ventilator system checks. Respiratory Care 37:884, 1992.

AARC: Clinical practice guideline: Ventilator circuit changes. Respiratory Care 39:800, 1994.

AARC: Clinical practice guideline: Fiberoptic bronchoscopy assisting. Respiratory Care 38:1173, 1993.

AARC: Clinical practice guideline: Long-term invasive mechanical ventilation in the home. Respiratory Care 40:1313, 1995.

American Heart Association: Guidelines for cardiopulmonary resuscitation and emergency cardiac care. JAMA 268:2213, 1992.

Hess, D and Ravikumar, A: Methods of emergency drug administration. Respiratory Care 40:503, 1995.

PRIORITIES

GENERAL

Vital signs
Responsiveness
ABG
Physical observation
Oximetry

AIRWAY

Check and maintain patency
Manage artificial airway
Provide airway care/suctioning

VENTILATION/OXYGENATION

Monitor and support ventilation (PPV)
Assure oxygenation
Monitor: ABG, auscultation, palpation, observation,
    percussion, airway pressure, MV settings
    and changes, patient responses

DIAGNOSTICS

CT scan
X-rays
EEG
ECG
Hemodynamics
Bronchoscopy
Lab. studies
? Angiography
Surgeries

CIRCULATION

Monitor: hemodynamics, urine output, capillary
    refill

NEUROLOGICAL RECOVERY

Motor response
Pupillary response
Cognitive response
Level of coma
ICP
Vision/focus

OTHER CONCERNS

Gastrointestinal problems
Renal complications
Musculoskeletal problems
Electrolyte balance
Infection control
Psychosocial development/training/support
Mobility/physical conditioning
Skin integrity
Rehabilitation/transition to other facility/home
Long-term planning
Equipment maintenance/safety/quality assurance
Communication

Figure 16–4. Concept map of the respiratory care of Elle Carey.

Kacmarek, R: Management of the patient-mechanical ventilator system. In: Kacmarek, R and Pierson, D: Foundations of Respiratory Care. Churchill Livingstone, New York, 1992, pp. 989–990.

Phillips, R and Feeney, M: The Cardiac Rhythms, ed 3. WB Saunders, Philadelphia, 1990.

Schenk, E: Management of persons with common neurologic manifestations. In: Phipps, W et al: Medical Surgical Nursing. Mosby, St. Louis, 1991, p. 1800.

Severinghaus, J: Role of cerebrospinal fluid pH in normalization of cerebral blood flow in chronic hypocapnia. Acta Neurol Scand 14:116–120, 1965.

Smeltzer, C and Bare, B: Brunner and Suddarth's Textbook of Medical-Surgical Nursing, ed 7. JB Lippincott, Philadelphia, 1992, p. 1739.

Stein, E: Clinical Electrocardiography. Lea & Febiger, Philadelphia, 1987.

PRACTICE QUESTIONS

1. During basic life support delivery, using a manual resuscitator for ventilation, the RCP sees that the victim's abdomen becomes markedly distended. The RCP should recommend:
   A. Compression of the abdomen
   B. A larger mask
   C. Increasing the source gas flow
   D. Endotracheal intubation
   E. Nasal suctioning

2. Signs associated with a tension pneumothorax include all of the following except:
   A. Absence of breath sounds over the affected area
   B. Tracheal deviation toward the affected area
   C. Lack of markings on CXR
   D. Increased inspiratory pressures
   E. A decrease in dynamic lung compliance

3. Interpret the following ECG and make a recommendation:

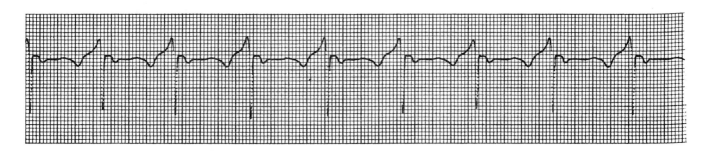

A. Do nothing.
B. Request lidocaine.
C. Administer atropine.
D. Deliver a precordial thump.
E. Defibrillate.

4. Evaluation of proper airway placement includes which of the following?
   I. End tidal carbon dioxide measurement
   II. Auscultation of breath sounds
   III. Chest x-ray
   IV. Pulse oximetry
   V. Passage of a suction catheter through the tube
      A. I, II, III, IV, and V
      B. I, III, and V
      C. II and IV
      D. I, II, III, and V
      E. II, III, and V

5. The first-line drug for the treatment of ventricular dysrhythmia in adults is:
   A. Atropine
   B. Oxygen
   C. Fentanyl
   D. Procainamide
   E. Lidocaine

6. Obtain a copy of the AARC Clinical Practice Guidelines. According to the guideline Patient-Ventilator System Checks, a ventilator check should be performed under all of the following circumstances except:
   A. Before ventilator circuit changes
   B. Following any change in settings
   C. Prior to obtaining blood gas samples
   D. Following an acute deterioration of the patient's condition, particularly when this occurs after violation of a ventilator alarm threshold
   E. At regularly scheduled intervals

7. In accordance with the AARC guideline Long-Term Invasive Mechanical Ventilation in the Home, contraindications include:
   I. Lack of an appropriate discharge plan
   II. $FIO_2 > 0.40$
   III. PEEP > 10 cm H_2O
   IV. Inadequate numbers of competent caregivers
   V. Inadequate financial resources
      A. I, II, and III
      B. I, II, III, IV, and V
      C. II and III
      D. I, IV, and V
      E. II, III, and IV

8. As part of the discharge planning team, the RCP should realize that the plan includes:
   A. Evaluation of the patient for the appropriateness of the discharge
   B. Determination of the optimal site of care and of patient care resources
   C. Determination that financial resources are adequate
   D. A and B
   E. A, B, and C

9. A blood sample used to measure the mixed venous partial pressure of oxygen would be sampled using:
   A. An arterial catheter
   B. An oxygen analyzer
   C. The proximal tip of the PA-catheter
   D. The distal tip of the PA-catheter
   E. The co-oximeter

10. Urine output is considered within the normal range if it is:
    A. 30 to 50 mL/h
    B. 60 to 90 mL/h
    C. 10 to 20 mL/h
    D. 20 to 30 mL/h
    E. >80 mL/h

17 | Mort Merten: An Infant with Meconium Aspiration Syndrome

Learning Objectives

After reading the chapter and performing the activities within it, the learner will be able to:

- Identify the risks and complications associated with meconium aspiration syndrome (MAS).
- Determine objectives, interventions, and evaluations for the care plan.
- Make an inference regarding quality assurance and improvement issues.
- Make recommendations regarding changes in the regimen.
- Perform trend analysis using available assessment data.
- Explain the rationale for the modalities used and the plans made.
- Use a systematic problem-solving approach to create a desired outcome.

Key Words and Phrases

Apgar
Cervical dilation
Chest drainage
Decelerations
Dubowitz
Effacement
Fetal heart rate (FHR)
Fetal scalp pH
  Gestation
Labor
Meconium
Meconium aspiration
  syndrome (MAS)

Pneumothorax
Preductal and postductal
Preeclampsia
Pregnancy-induced
  hypertension (PIH)
Primigravida
Rupture of the membranes
  (ROM)
Transcutaneous monitoring
  (TCM)

INTRODUCTION

The case presented represents the potential course of events surrounding the birth of a 44-week-*gestation* male baby, Mort Merten. Remember, not all case details are included, and the use of Figures 1 through 3 and varied resources will enrich the learning experience.

DELIVERY ROOM

A 24-year-old *primigravida* presents in stage 2 of *labor*, after 20 hours in stage 1. The high-risk delivery team is assembled. Labor history is as follows:

RCP notation.
Day 2: 2:28 AM
The patient presented with her husband as birthing partner at 12:30 PM yesterday.

PMH is not significant for medical problems.
Approximate gestation is 43 wk.
Rupture of membranes (ROM) occurred at home.
Presence of *meconium* is confirmed and is noted to be thick, +4. (*Scale is 1–4, with 1 being least or little and 4 being most or thickest.*)
Vaginal bleeding noted upon admission.
Maternal BP = 180/116 (baseline has been 138/87). HR = 165 (sinus).
Peripheral edema noted. Hyperreflexia noted. Urine protein = 4+ (*loss of 5 g or more over 24 h*).
BS are clear to auscultation and percussion.
Fetal heart rate (FHR) (baseline) is 120–138 with late *decelerations* lasting approximately 120 s.
FHR has maintained short-term variability.
Fetal scalp pH = 7.26.

Uterine contractions (UC) occur q 1 min, lasting 160 s and strong.

Mother has been maintained mostly in the left side-lying position.

Cervical dilation is 9 cm with the fetus in station +5, right occiput anterior presentation (ROA), 100% *effacement*.

⇨ Thought Prompts

1. Assess the factors that place the fetus at risk for physical problems.
2. What risks are present for the mother?
3. Do the maternal assessment data illustrate a particular problem?
4. Analyze the data for the fetus and determine whether asphyxia is likely to have occurred.
5. What is indicated by the late decelerations of the fetal heart?
6. As the RCP, what preparations should be made at this time?
7. Devise an action plan for the delivery. Be sure to note the evaluations you would use in a situation like this.

DELIVERY

The vaginal birth is uncomplicated as stage 2 concludes with birth. The mother is stable with IV magnesium sulfate infusing at present and 100% oxygen being delivered by a nonrebreathing (NRB) oxygen mask. As the head of the infant presents, meconium is noted on the skin, in the oral cavity, and in the oropharynx.

⇨ Thought Prompts

8. Should any intervention occur at this point? If so, what?
9. Identify the indication and action of magnesium sulfate in this case.

Clinical Notations: Admission

Values not listed may be considered insignificant at this point.

General Care	RC Assessments	RC Interventions	Recom-mendations
Admission to labor and delivery (L&D)	ROM. Vaginal bleeding (moderate). Meconium present (+4). 43-wk gestation. Maternal BP = 180/116. HR = 165. Peripheral edema noted. Clear chest exam.	100% nonbreathing mask applied to mother.	Prepare for high-risk delivery. Assemble and check resuscitation equipment. Prepare radiant warmer.

Mild dyspnea with labor.
FHR = 120–138 with late decelerations, lasting 120 s.
Short-term variability noted.
Fetal scalp pH = 7.26, checked × 2.
UC q 1 min × 160 s, strong.
Fully dilated, effaced 100%, station +5, ROA.
Mother is alert and cooperative.

Delivery	Mother stable with MgSO₄ IV. 100% O₂.	Gathered, checked, and assembled suction equipment. Resuscitation supplies and warmer ready for use.	Prepare for tracheal suction prior to delivery of the fetal shoulders.

FHR = fetal heart rate, MgSO₄ = magnesium sulfate, ROA = right occiput anterior (position of fetus), ROM = rupture of membranes, UC = uterine contractions.

⇨ Thought Prompts

10. Explain the process for assembling and checking suction equipment.
11. Describe the suctioning procedure indicated at this point.
12. What is the rationale for suctioning the meconium prior to delivery of the fetal body?
13. What supplies must the RCP assemble and check prior to resuscitation?
14. Discuss the policies and procedures associated with maintaining readiness for emergency situations like the one described in this chapter. Are systems in place to maintain readiness on a continuous basis? If not, can you create such a system?

Clinical Notations: Postpartum, Delivery Room

General Care	RC Assessments	RC Interventions	Recom-mendations
Postpartum phase in delivery room	Infant wt. = 4.0 kg. Mother remains stable and is attended by nurse. Infant *Apgar* is 3 at 1 min. After 30 s of PPV, HR = 30 bpm.	Neonatal resuscitation instituted. Chest compressions continued.	Institute resuscitation.

⇨ Thought Prompts

15. Using Figure 17–1, identify and discuss the relevance of the initial steps outlined (e.g., warming, drying, and stimulating).

Overview of Resuscitation in the Delivery Room

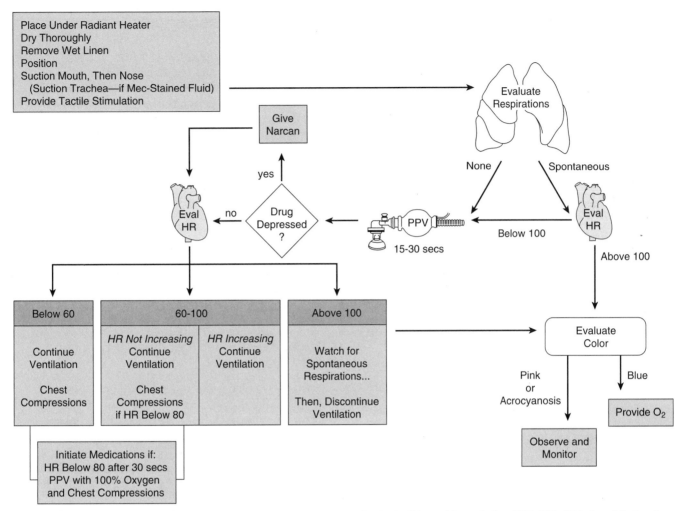

Figure 17–1. Overview of neonatal resuscitation. (Reproduced with permission. Textbook of Neonatal Resuscitation, 1987, 1990, 1994. Copyright American Heart Association.)

16. Using Table 17–1 as a reference, create a scenario that would lead to an infant's having an Apgar score of 3. (Many possibilities exist.)
17. What type of hand resuscitator is used on the neonate, and how is it monitored?
18. What evaluations are used to assess the neonate being resuscitated?
19. Is it preferable to bag-mask-ventilate this infant, or is intubation with an endotracheal tube preferred? Why?
20. What anatomical features of the neonate present difficulties for intubation?
21. Explain the procedure for intubation of the neonate.
22. What type and size of artificial airway are indicated?
23. How may tube placement be assessed?

Table 17–1	APGAR SCORING SYSTEM		
Value	0	1	2
Heart rate	None	<100 bpm	>100 bpm
Respiratory rate	None	Weak, irregular	Strong cry
Color	Pale, blue	Body pink, extremities blue	Completely pink
Reflex	No response	Grimace	Cry, cough
Muscle tone	Limp	Some flexion	Well flexed

Clinical Notations: Postpartum, Transport to Neonatal Intensive Care Unit

Mort Merten is stabilized in the delivery room and transported to the NICU, where he is placed on PPV via a mechanical time-cycled, pressure-limited ventilator. His mother is recovering in the postpartum unit. His father is in conference with the neonatal fellow on the case.

⇨ Thought Prompts

24. In what ways will the RCP in this case, now transporting the infant, require collaboration from fellow health care workers?
25. Describe how the practitioner could manage the infant's transport, NICU preparations, and NICU admission assessments.

Clinical Notations: Admission to Neonatal Intensive Care Unit

General Care	RC Assessments	RC Interventions	Recom- mendations
NICU admission	Gestational age = 44 wk by *Dubowitz* scoring. Wt. = 4.0 kg. Ht. = 22 in. Growth, including head, is appropriate for gestational age. Physical exam: Peripheral cyanosis. Alert and moving all extremities. Reflexes are normal. HR = 165, sinus rhythm. No murmurs detected. BP = 70/40 SpO_2 > 96% by oximetry, right earlobe. Asymmetrical chest expansion noted, with left side not expanding as fully as right. UAC is placed with ABGs: PaO_2 = 40 $PaCO_2$ = 50 pH = 7.31 HCO_3^- = 24 SaO_2 = 75% Retractions present. Nasal flaring noted. BS reveal coarse crackles over RUL and RML with clear BS over RLL. BS over left chest are not heard. STAT CXR ordered.	Hand resuscitation with 50% via non-self-inflating bag, with PPV RR of 60–70 and PAWP @ 40 cm/5 cm PEEP, with I:E @ 1:1 has been maintained. Ventilator attached @ same settings used in hand resuscitation. TCM initiated.	Prepare trans-illumination equipment. Gather, assemble, and check TCM unit. Assess and treat per RC NICU protocol.

ht. = height, I:E = inspiratory to expiratory ratio, PAWP = peak airway pressure, PEEP = positive end expiratory pressure, PPV = positive pressure ventilation, RML = right middle lobe, RUL = right upper lobe, TCM = transcutaneous monitor, UAC = umbilical artery catheter, wt. = weight.

⇨ Thought Prompts

26. What associated problem is likely to have occurred now?
27. What assessments support your conclusion?
28. Discuss other assessments that may give additional confirming data.
29. What intervention is indicated at this point?

30. Present an argument for using short inspiratory times in the case of *meconium aspiration syndrome (MAS)*.
31. Interpret the ABGs.
32. Analyze the situation and make recommendations regarding PPV.
33. Describe the effect that increasing the PEEP would have on ventilation.
34. Describe the process of transillumination and identify its indication in this case.
35. Explain the process of checking the function of a *transcutaneous monitor (TCM)*.
36. What quality assurance measures should be performed routinely on the TCM?
37. How often should probe sites be changed?
38. What assessments would indicate the need to change probe sites sooner?
39. What are desirable locations for TCM probe sites?

Clinical Notations: Neonatal Intensive Care Unit, Day 1

General Care	RC Assessments	RC Interventions	Recom- mendations
NICU, day 1	Presence of left apical *pneumothorax* confirmed by transillumination, then by CXR and percussion.	Gather, assemble, and check pulmonary drainage unit.	

⇨ Thought Prompts

40. Create the RC plan for the case up to this point.

Objectives:	Inter- ventions:	Indications/ rationales:	Evalu- ations:
1. Assure ventilation:			
2. Assure oxygenation:			
3. Maintain airway patency:			
4. Prevent infection:			
5. Promote patient safety:			

41. Label the diagram on the opposite page, and note the function of each component. Explain how this unit's operation is verified. (Label the parts A, B, and C.)

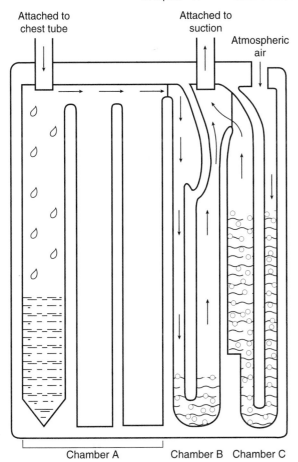

Attached to chest tube

Attached to suction

Atmospheric air

Chamber A   Chamber B Chamber C

Clinical Notations: Neonatal Intensive Care Unit, Days 1 and 2

General Care	RC Assessments	RC Interventions	Recom-mendations
NICU, day 1	Chest tube inserted by physician in left apical chest. BS improving. Chest expansion is more symmetrical. Ventilator settings remain unchanged. Color is improved. Flaring and retractions are absent. ABGs @ present on 50%. FIO_2/PAWP @ 45 cm H_2O with PEEP of 5 cm H_2O. PaO_2 = 72 $PaCO_2$ = 45 pH = 7.35 HCO_3^- = 23 from UAC. VS are unchanged. CXR repeated.	Connect to pulmonary drainage unit.	Monitor patient and drainage unit q 1 h this shift. Follow RC plan.
Day 2	*Preductal and postductal* TCM values for $PtcO_2$ show a 40-mm Hg gradient.		Continue plan. Consult with neonatologist and primary nurse regarding findings.

Thought Prompts

42. How would you classify Mort Merten's response to *chest drainage* tube insertion?
43. What is indicated by the preductal and postductal gradient identified by TCM?
44. If ventilatory and oxygen demands could not be satisfied and the patient were not responding to conventional ventilation, what other possible therapeutic modalities would be available for treatment?
45. Describe some of the risks and benefits of the following options:
    Extracorporeal membrane oxygenation (ECMO):

    PPV with nitric oxide:

    High-frequency ventilation:

Clinical Notations: Neonatal Intensive Care Unit, Days 3 through 5

Over the next 3 days Mort Merten stabilizes and weans from PPV. He is treated with tolazoline with good results. He is assessed as not needing supplemental oxygen at this point and is being admitted to the special care nursery. Chest drainage is discontinued with full resolution of the pneumothorax. CXR reveals a small infiltrate in the RUL. His mother has been having seizures and is in coma. His father has had several outbursts in the NICU, showing much anger toward the staff.

Thought Prompts

46. In what ways can the RCP promote effective coping strategies in the father of this newborn and in the RCP himself or herself?
47. Adjust the RC plan to Mort Merten's current condition. Be sure to assess all potential risks.
48. Obtain a copy of the AARC Clinical Practice Guidelines. Identify the CPGs that would be valuable resources in working through this case.

Bibliography

Barnhart, S and Czervinske, M: Clinical Handbook of Perinatal and Pediatric Respiratory Care. WB Saunders, Philadelphia, 1995.

Olds, S, London, M and Ladewig, P: Maternal Newborn Nursing, ed 4. Addison-Wesley, Redwood, CA, 1992.

Smith-Wenning, K et al: Neonatal and Pediatric Respiratory Care. In: Scanlan, C: Egan's Fundamentals of Respiratory Care. Mosby, St. Louis, 1995.

Whittaker, K: Comprehensive Perinatal and Pediatric Respiratory Care. Delmar, Albany, NY, 1992.

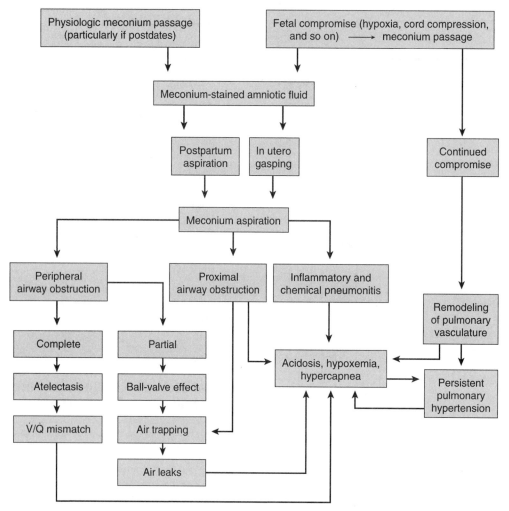

Figure 17–2. Pathophysiology of the passage of meconium and the meconium aspiration syndrome. (Adapted from Bacsik, RD: Meconium aspiration syndrome. Pediatr Clin North Am 24:467, 1977.)

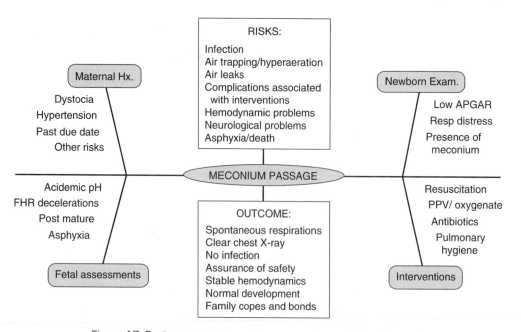

Figure 17–3. Concept map summarizing assessments associated with meconium passage.

PRACTICE QUESTIONS

1. All of the following describe the neonatal airway except:
   A. It has a relatively large tongue.
   B. The narrowest part is the cricoid ring.
   C. The epiglottis lies horizontally.
   D. It has a very compliant chest wall.
   E. The trachea is 11 cm in length.

2. When the RCP suctions a nasally intubated neonate who has a size 3.0-mm endotracheal tube in place, respiratory distress is noted. To correct this, the RCP should:
   A. Change to a larger suction catheter.
   B. Hyperoxygenate before the procedure.
   C. Call the physician STAT.
   D. Request an ABG.
   E. Request a CXR.

3. The CXR associated with meconium aspiration syndrome will likely reflect:
   A. Miliary lesions
   B. Fibrotic changes
   C. Mycetomas
   D. Bronchospasm
   E. Hyperinflation

4. Which of the following represent suctioning complications in the neonate?
   I. Infection
   II. Atelectasis
   III. Increased BP
   IV. Bradycardia
   V. Pneumothorax
      A. I, II, III, IV, and V
      B. II and V
      C. I, II, IV, and V
      D. II, III, and V
      E. I, III, and V

5. When a neonate is being resuscitated in the delivery room and he or she is found to have a heart rate of 40 bpm without spontaneous respirations, what should be done?
   A. Administer epinephrine.
   B. Administer oxygen.
   C. Give chest compressions.
   D. Perform mechanical ventilations.
   E. Both C and D.

6. A 2400-g neonate intubated and mechanically ventilated with a time-cycled ventilator presents with the following:

ABGs: WBC: CXR:
   $PaO_2 = 70$ 25,000   RLL pneumonia
   $PaCO_2 = 78$
   $pH = 7.07$
   $HCO_3^- = 24$

Which of the following should occur first?
   A. Increase the set tidal volume.
   B. Administer antibiotics.
   C. Deliver chest physiotherapy.
   D. Increase the set peak airway pressure (cycling pressure).
   E. Decrease the respiratory rate.

7. Which of the following best describes high-frequency oscillation?
   A. Delivery of short breaths via a triple-lumen endotracheal tube
   B. Delivery of extremely small breaths, generated by a piston speaker, including active expiration
   C. High rates of conventional ventilation
   D. Delivery of short, high-pressure breaths administered proximal to the ETT
   E. Delivery of high rates of ventilation incorporating less than dead space volumes

8. Given an I:E ratio of 1:2 and a respiratory rate of 30, calculate the inspiratory time.
   A. 0.7 s
   B. 1 s
   C. 2 s
   D. 0.2 s
   E. Not enough information to solve

9. Maintenance of a pulmonary drainage unit commonly includes:
   A. Stripping or milking of the tubes
   B. Disconnecting the tube from the unit for pulmonary hygiene routines
   C. Administering medication via the atmospheric port
   D. Monitoring the volume of fluid in the chambers
   E. Applying 50 to 70 cm H_2O of suction pressure for drainage

10. To drain an empyema, the chest tube should be inserted in:
   A. The sixth or seventh interspace in the midaxillary or posterior axillary line
   B. The third or fourth interspace in the midaxillary line
   C. The apex of the pleural space
   D. The pericardium
   E. The diaphragmatic space

18 | Kyle Hicks: An Infant with Respiratory Distress Syndrome

Learning Objectives

After reading the chapter and performing the activities within it, the learner will be able to:

- Recognize assessment data pertaining to the problem of respiratory distress syndrome (RDS).
- Identify indications, interventions, objectives, and expected outcomes related to the RC plan.
- Identify the initial sequence of events in neonatal resuscitation.
- Select an appropriate monitoring plan for the case.
- Determine positive versus negative responses to interventions in the case.
- Integrate into the case the following AARC CPGs by using them to develop the RC plan: Oximetry, Patient-Ventilator System Checks, Circuit Changes; Endotracheal Suctioning; Oxygen Therapy in the Acute Care Setting; Oxygen Therapy in the Homecare Setting; Transcutaneous Monitoring; Neonatal Mechanical Ventilation; Application of CPAP; Resuscitation in Acute Care Hospitals; Surfactant Replacement Therapy; and Capillary Blood Gas Sampling for Neonatal and Pediatric Patients.

Key Words and Phrases

Apgar
Cesarean-section delivery (C-section)
Dubowitz scoring system
Fetal heart decelerations
Grunting, retractions
Guaiac-positive
Lecithin/sphingomyelin (L/S) ratio
Maternal risk factors

Nasopharyngeal CPAP (NP-CPAP)
Neonatal resuscitation
Primigravida
Respiratory distress syndrome (RDS)
Surfactant
Thermoregulation
Tocolysis
Transcutaneous monitoring (TCM)

INTRODUCTION

This case follows the progress of a neonatal patient, Kyle Hicks. The learner is encouraged to stimulate discussion and use multiple resources (see bibliography at the chapter's end) in the study of this case in RC. (Note: The notations represent only part of the medical record.)

ADMISSION NOTE

This 1020-g boy, twin B, was delivered by *cesarean section (C-section)* at 8:05 AM. His brother, twin A, weighing 1339 g,

was delivered about 5 minutes earlier. *Dubowitz* scoring determines gestational age to be 29 weeks.

Maternal History

Mother is a 15-year-old *primigravida.*
Positive for mild gestational diabetes.
Received prenatal care.
Has parental support. Her mother attended the delivery.
Other information found in obstetric history represents normal findings.

Labor and Delivery

Received terbutaline for *tocolysis*. Negative response.

During stage 1 of labor, type II *fetal heart decelerations* were noted. Fetal scalp pH of twin A was 7.20 at this time.

Decision to perform C-section confirmed.

BP unrecognizable. Doppler used.
Central cyanosis noted.
Extremities were flaccid.
No response to stimuli noted.
L/S (lecithin/sphingomyelin) ratio = 1
Surfactant replacement therapy is initiated, as is *resuscitation*.

⇨ **Thought Prompts**

1. Using resources within this text and others, list the assessed factors that indicate that lung maturation of twin B may be decelerated. (*Note:* You may need to define several terms in the preceding section to understand the assessment data.)
2. What *maternal risk factors* contribute to the fetal condition?
3. What was the purpose of terbutaline administration? Can you list other medications that can be used for this purpose?
4. Describe the significance of the fetal heart decelerations and the scalp pH. Does a relationship exist between the two? (Do they indicate the same problem?)

⇨ **Thought Prompts**

5. Discuss the data that indicate *respiratory distress syndrome (RDS)* as the diagnosis.
6. Compute the *Apgar* score for this infant (use Table 17–1).
7. Using Figure 17–1, record the sequence of neonatal resuscitation that should take place. You may include medications and dosages or, if time does not permit, you may simply outline the steps of resuscitation.
8. Determine the following:
   Appropriate size of oral endotracheal tube for this infant: _____
   Types of commercially available surfactant:

   _____

   _____

   Surfactant administration technique:

9. What indications are present for surfactant replacement therapy?

10. Fill in the following map about exogenous surfactant. Fill in at the places marked with an asterisk. Place an arrow indicating increase or decrease (↑ or ↓) or write the correct phrase.

Labor and Delivery (*Continued*)

Neonatal resuscitation teams were called.

Twins A and B were delivered, C-section (no delivery or surgical complications occurred). The following notations are specific for twin B.

Available Assessments

HR = 20 bpm.
RR = 0.

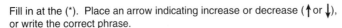

Fill in at the (*). Place an arrow indicating increase or decrease (↑ or ↓), or write the correct phrase.

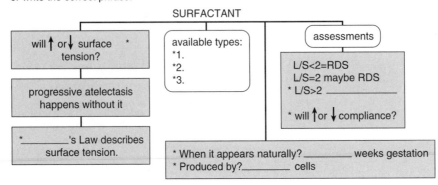

NURSING NOTE

Nursing Diagnoses

Impaired gas exchange: Related to RDS
Ineffective thermoregulation: Related to prematurity
Ineffective airway clearance: Related to artificial airway
Potential for infection: Related to gestational age
Altered nutrition: Related to prematurity
Altered family process: Related to hospitalization

Patient Outcomes

ABGs are within normal limits.
Cold stress is prevented.
Airway patency is maintained.
Patient demonstrates absence of infection.
Patient tolerates feeding.
Family demonstrates bonding by taking on infant care
duties.

RESPIRATORY CARE NEONATAL INTENSIVE CARE UNIT ADMISSION NOTE

Baby Hicks, twin B, is admitted to NICU at 8:25 AM. Was transported from delivery room, via transport incubator, on 5 cm H_2O *nasopharyngeal CPAP (NP-CPAP)*, with size 3.0 nasopharyngeal tube. No significant events ensued during transport. FIO_2 is 0.40 at present.

Significant Clinical Data

RR = 34	PaO_2 = 58	WBC = 25,000/mm³
(spontaneous)	$PaCO_2$ = 43	RBC = 4.0 mil/mm³
HR = 165	pH = 7.36	Hct = 48%
BP = 44/28	HCO_3^- = 22	Hgb = 15 g/dL
Na = 139	SpO_2 = 92%	
K = 5.5		
Serum glucose =		
28 mg/dL		

RESPIRATORY CARE PLAN

Indications for Respiratory Care

1. Oxygen and humidity deficit
2. Apnea of prematurity
3. RDS
4. Artificial airway in place
5. Immature *thermoregulation* mechanisms
6. Inability to maintain self-care

Objectives

1. Maintain PaO_2 between 50 and 90 mm Hg.
2. Maintain $PaCO_2$ between 35 and 45, with pH between 7.35 and 7.45.
3. Prevent progression of RDS/atelectasis.
4. Prevent secretion retention and maintain airway patency.
5. Prevent conductive, convective, radiation, and evaporative heat loss.
6. Optimize patient safety.

Interventions

1. Oxygenation @ 40% FIO_2 with NP-CPAP of 5 cm H_2O. Progressively wean to oxyhood, then cannula if needed. Provide 100% warmed humidity.
2. Monitor ventilation status, *stimulate,* and *assist* when indicated.
3. Implement bronchial hygiene protocol (hyperinflation, percussion, vibration).
4. Perform airway care prn.
5. Maintain neutral thermal environment. Monitor inspired gas.

Monitor

Transcutaneous blood gas monitoring (continuous).
ABGs as indicated by protocol.
Oximetry (continuous).
CXR as per protocol.
ECG (continuous).
Glucose testing as per protocol.
Patient-ventilator system checks q 2 h.
Temperatures: Skin, inspired, core, TC probe.
Monitor VS, color, activity, q 2 h.
Reevaluate plan q 24 h and update at NICU rounds.

Expected Outcomes

- Oxygenation and ventilation are adequate during spontaneous breathing.
- BS improve.
- CXR improves.
- VS are stable.
- Hemodynamics are stable.
- Body temperature is maintained and stable.
- Sputum production is minimal and maintained by patient crying and deep breathing.

⇨ **Thought Prompts**

11. What indications are present for the use of NP-CPAP?

12. Discuss the relationships among the five intervention strategies and the expected outcomes.
13. What assessments will be made to evaluate the achievement of the therapeutic objectives?
14. Describe positive responses to the interventions.
15. What negative responses could occur?
16. How can conductive, convective, radiation, and evaporative heat loss be prevented?
17. Explain why *transcutaneous monitoring (TCM)* is performed on a continuous basis rather than on a spot-check schedule.
18. Discuss the components of performing airway care on this infant.
19. Is the plan complete and appropriate?

Clinical Notations: Days 1 and 2

Day	General Care	RC Assessments	RC Interventions	Recommendations
Day 1, 8:05 AM	Resuscitation . . . Hydration Labs/electrolytes WBC = 28,000/ mm^3 Surfactant replacement	HR < 50. Respirations absent. Flaccid posture. Nonresponsive. Central cyanosis. Very low birth weight (1020 g). 29 wk gestation. L/S = 1	Intubate and PPV. Oxygenate. Warm, dry, and stimulate.	Follow neonatal resuscitation guidelines. Follow surfactant administration protocol.
8:25 AM, NICU	Transfer to NICU IV access UAC line	PaO$_2$ = 58. PaCO$_2$ = 43. pH = 7.36. HCO$_3^-$ = 22. SpO$_2$ = 92% (on CPAP of 5 and 40 % O$_2$). HR = 165. RR = 34 (spontaneous). BP = 44/28.	NP-CPAP 5 cm and 40% FIO$_2$	Follow RC plan. CPAP system checks q 2 h.
2:00 PM	Maintain	*Grunting. Retractions.* Nasal flaring. PaO$_2$ = 50. PaCO$_2$ = 47. pH = 7.34. HCO$_3^-$ = 21. Coarse BS bilat. CXR = ground glass.	Begin PPV with time-cycled, pressure-limited vent. PIP = 18 cm H$_2$O. PEEP = 5. FIO$_2$ = 45%. RR = 35. IT = 0.57 s. I:E ratio = 1:2. Mode: SIMV.	Initiate PPV system checks q 2 h. Monitor cardiopulm status continuously (ECG, RR, etc.).

Baby Hicks remains stable throughout the 3:00 PM to 11:00 PM shift.

Day	General Care	RC Assessments	RC Interventions	Recommendations
Day 2, 12:15 AM	*Guaiac-positive* stools. Abdominal distention noted. WBC = 36,000/ mm^3.	PaO$_2$ = 49. PaCO$_2$ = 45. pH = 7.34. HCO$_3^-$ = 20.	↑FIO$_2$ to 50%. Maintain other settings.	Improve oxygenation.
1:00 AM	NG suction. NPO. Gentamicin started. Abdominal x-ray reveals gas bubbles in the intestinal wall.	PaO$_2$ = 50. (Acid-base WNL.)	No changes. Reposition endotube. Clean mouth.	Follow current plan. Meet O$_2$ demand. Begin TCM. Change TC probe site q 3 h.
1:25 AM	VS stable. Lethargy noted.	PtcO$_2$ = 54.	TCM.	Maintain plan. Begin CPT in AM q 3 h before feeding.

Baby Hicks has few episodes of desaturation and dropping PtcO$_2$ . . . but remains essentially stable throughout the rest of day 2.

⇨ **Thought Prompts**

20. What indicates the introduction of PPV into the case on Day 1?
21. Describe time-triggered, pressure-limited, time-cycled mechanical ventilation.
22. Are the ventilator settings appropriate for the circumstance?
23. On Day 2 what significant assessments are noted?
24. What condition is described by these assessments?
25. Describe the relationship between the condition in the preceding question and the increased oxygen demand that occurred at the same time.

Clinical Notations: Days 3 and 4

Day	General Care	RC Assessments	RC Interventions	Recommendations
Day 3, 6:00 AM	Mild cardiac murmur noted.	PtcO$_2$ = 79 (R chest) PtcO$_2$ = 55 (abdomen)		Begin weaning RR. Suggest indomethacin (request denied).
10:00 AM	Stable. Crying more robustly.	Same	MV RR ↓ to 30	Continue to wean.
10:20 AM		PaO$_2$ = 53 PaCO$_2$ = 45 pH = 7.35 RR (spontaneous) = 15	MV RR ↓ to 25	

Baby Hicks maintains acid-base balance with decreasing PPV as the day progresses. RR is decreased to 14 by 8:00 PM and then FIO$_2$ is decreased to 45% with PaO$_2$ = 52.

Day	General Care	RC Assessments	RC Interventions	Recommendations
Day 4, 5:00 AM, PPV	Stable. Abdominal x-ray improved.	Spont RR = 25 PtcO$_2$ = 51 (R chest) PtcO$_2$ = 49 (abdomen) CXR = opaque densities throughout	MMV RR ↓ to 10	Wean. Reinstitute CPAP of 5 cm H$_2$O and 45% FIO$_2$.

Baby Hicks continues to wean from PPV and is placed on CPAP when PPV rate is decreased to 4.

⇨ **Thought Prompts**

26. On Day 3 what do the cardiac murmur and PtcO$_2$ gradient (described) indicate?
27. Why was indomethacin requested on Day 3? Why was the request denied?
28. Using the data available, determine whether the progression of ventilator weaning started on Day 3 was appropriate.
29. Create therapeutic objectives for the RC weaning plan. (State objectives in terms of outcome.)

Clinical Notations:
Days 5, 8, 20, and 30

Day	General Care	RC Assessments	RC Interventions	Recommendations
Day 5	NG suction. d/c'd	Spont RR = 38. ABGs in safe range.	CPAP of 5 with 45% FiO_2	

Baby Hicks remains stable but oxygen requirements are still high. CPAP and FiO_2 weaned slowly.

Day	General Care	RC Assessments	RC Interventions	Recommendations
Day 8	VS stable.	$PaO_2 = 50$. $PaCO_2 = 42$. pH = 7.40. $HCO_3^- = 21$ mEq/dL.	On CPAP = 4 cm H_2O and 30% FiO_2	Extubate. Institute O_2 therapy via oxyhood.

Baby Hicks adapts to heated and humidified oxyhood and FiO_2 is slowly decreased.

Day	General Care	RC Assessments	RC Interventions	Recommendations
Day 20	VS stable.	ABGs within safe range. BS reveal wheezing bilat. CXR reveals cystic formation throughout. Is suctioned nasally on average of × 4 per day for 6–10 mL sputum total production.	On nasal cannula @ 0.6 L/min	Maintain O_2 status. Begin broncho-dilator therapy.
Day 30	Discharge planned.	CXR reveals large cystic lesions. ABGs on 21%: $PaO_2 = 48$ $PaCO_2 = 44$ pH = 7.39 $HCO_3^- = 22$ ABGs on nasal cannula @ 0.41/min: $PaO_2 = 55$ $PaCO_2 = 43$ pH = 7.39 $HCO_3^- = 22$ Baby Hicks active, moving all limbs appropriately. VS are stable.		Home therapy: Oxygen via cannula @ 0.4 L/min. Bronchodilator aerosol therapy q 6 h. Parental instruction and educa-tion. Ongoing assessment.

CPT = chest physiotherapy, HR = heart rate, L/S = lecithin/sphingomyelin ratio, NG = nasogastric, NP-CPAP = nasopharyngeal continuous positive airway pressure, UAC = umbilical artery catheter, WBC = white blood count, WNL = within normal limits.

⇨ **Thought Prompts**

30. Examine the progression of Baby Hicks between Days 4 and 30. What is the likely diagnosis on discharge?
31. What are the indications for home therapy?
32. Considering the age and condition of this child, how do you suggest the oxygenation and ventilation status be assessed on an outpatient basis?
33. Given the case data, create a home RC plan for Kyle Hicks. Be sure to include an evaluation and monitoring plan and specify the expected outcome.

Bibliography

AARC: Clinical practice guideline: Pulse oximetry. Respiratory Care 36:1406, 1991.

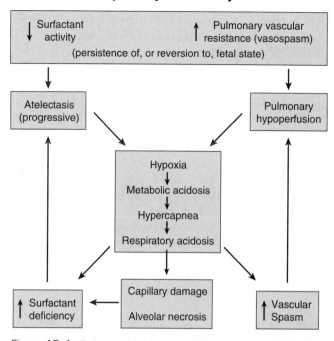

Figure 18–1. Pathogenesis of respiratory distress syndrome (RDS). (Reproduced by permission. Comprehensive Perinatal and Pediatric Respiratory Care by K. Whitaker. Delmar Publishers, Albany, NY, Copyright 1992, p. 352.)

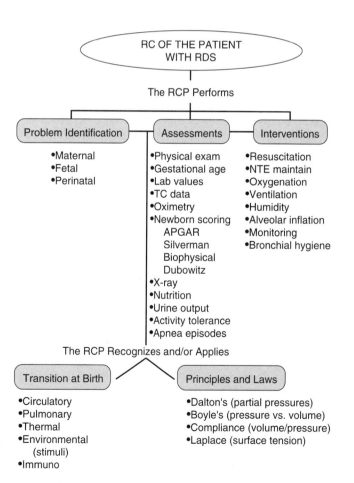

Figure 18–2. Learning issues in the case of Kyle Hicks.

AARC: Clinical practice guideline: Oxygen therapy in the acute care hospital. Respiratory Care 36:1410, 1991.

AARC: Clinical practice guideline: Patient ventilator system checks. Respiratory Care 37:882, 1992.

AARC: Clinical practice guideline: Oxygen therapy in the home or extended care facility. Respiratory Care 37:918, 1992.

AARC: Clinical practice guideline: Endotracheal suctioning of mechanically ventilated adults and children with artificial airways. Respiratory Care 38:500, 1993.

AARC: Clinical practice guideline: Resuscitation in acute care hospitals. Respiratory Care 38:1179, 1993.

AARC: Clinical practice guideline: Neonatal time-triggered, pressure-limited, time-cycled mechanical ventilation. Respiratory Care 39:808, 1994.

AARC: Clinical practice guideline: Surfactant replacement therapy. Respiratory Care 39:824, 1994.

AARC: Clinical practice guideline: Transcutaneous blood gas monitoring. Respiratory Care 39:1176, 1994.

Aloan, CA: Respiratory Care of the Newborn: A Clinical Manual. JB Lippincott, Philadelphia, 1987.

Barnhart, S and Czervinske, MP: Perinatal and Pediatric Respiratory Care. WB Saunders, Philadelphia, 1995.

Bloom, RS and Cropley, C: Textbook of Neonatal Resuscitation. American Heart Association/American Academy of Pediatrics, Dallas, 1987.

DesJardins, T: Clinical Manifestations and Assessment of Respiratory Disease, ed 3. Mosby-Year Book, St. Louis, 1995.

Farzan, S: A Concise Handbook of Respiratory Disease, ed 3. Appleton & Lange, Stamford, CT, 1992.

Kacmarek, R and Pierson, D: Foundations of Respiratory Care. Churchill-Livingstone, New York, 1992.

Koff, PB, Eitzman, DV and Neu, J: Neonatal and Pediatric Respiratory Care. CV Mosby, St. Louis, 1988.

Levin, D, Morriss, F and Moore, GC: A Practical Guide to Pediatric Intensive Care. CV Mosby, St. Louis, 1984.

Scanlan, C, Spearman, C and Sheldon, R: Egan's Fundamentals of Respiratory Care, ed 6. Mosby, St. Louis, 1995.

Whitaker, K: Comprehensive Perinatal and Pediatric Respiratory Care. Delmar, Albany, NY, 1992.

Wilkins, RL and Dexter, JR: Respiratory Disease: A Case Study Approach to Patient Care, ed 2. FA Davis, Philadelphia, 1997.

PRACTICE QUESTIONS

1. Complications associated with transport of the intubated neonate receiving CPAP may include:
   I. Hyperventilation related to manual ventilation
   II. Hemodynamic changes
   III. Accidental extubation
   IV. Disconnection from CPAP source
   V. Accidental removal of vascular access
      A. I, II, III, and V
      B. I, III, IV, and V
      C. II, III, IV, and V
      D. I, II, III, IV, and V
      E. I, III, and V

2. All of the following are limitations to the use of pulse oximetry except:
   A. Motion artifact
   B. Low perfusion states
   C. Skin pigmentation
   D. Abnormal hemoglobins
   E. Hyperbilirubinemia

3. Initial steps in neonatal resuscitation are:
   I. Place infant in radiant warmer.
   II. Provide 100% oxygen via hand resuscitator.
   III. Dry the infant.
   IV. Place the infant in the supine position and open the airway.
   V. Bulb-suction the nares and mouth.
      A. I, II, III, IV, and V
      B. I, III, IV, and V
      C. II, III, IV, and V
      D. I, III, and V
      E. II, III, and IV

4. Which of the following should be documented during TCM?
   A. The date and time of measurement.
   B. Inspired oxygen concentration or oxygen flow.
   C. Ventilator or CPAP data.
   D. Electrode placement site.
   E. All of these should be recorded.

5. Oxygen in the home care setting is indicated when:
   A. PaO_2 < 85 mm Hg in subjects breathing supplemental oxygen.
   B. $PaCO_2$ > 55 mm Hg.
   C. SaO_2 < 85% in subjects breathing room air.
   D. Hypoxemia and anemia are documented.
   E. Chronic pulmonary disease is diagnosed.

6. Which of the following reveals the highest maternal risk for fetal development?
   A. A 27-year-old obese woman
   B. A 15-year-old diabetic
   C. A 34-year-old in good health
   D. A 30-year-old with history of asthma
   E. A 26-year-old primigravida

7. An infant is delivered at 32 weeks' gestation. The following are recorded: HR is 80, feet and hands are cyanotic, and respirations are wheezy and at a rate of 35/min. The child is crying while moving the limbs about. Compute the Apgar score.
   A. 4
   B. 8
   C. 6
   D. 5
   E. 10

8. Which of the following types of fetal heart decelerations does *not* (or do not) indicate fetal hypoxia?
   A. Type I
   B. Type II
   C. Type III
   D. Types II and III
   E. Types I and II

9. All of the following are currently used to administer CPAP to the neonate except:
   A. Nasal prongs
   B. Nasopharyngeal tubes
   C. Endotracheal tubes
   D. Oxyhoods
   E. Tracheostomy tubes

10. Respiratory distress syndrome (RDS) is generally associated with:
   A. A patent ductus venosus
   B. Aspiration of meconium
   C. High-birth-weight neonates
   D. Low-birth-weight neonates
   E. Cesarean deliveries

19 | Eliza Hayes: A Burn Victim with Smoke Inhalation

Learning Objectives

After reading the chapter and performing the activities within it, the learner will be able to:

- Analyze the case data and form correct interpretations.
- Make sound evaluations based on case data.
- Regulate the RC plan as the case unfolds.
- Project acceptable outcomes for the plan.
- Perform self-evaluation and create self-objectives.

Key Words and Phrases

Bag-valve-mask (BVM) ventilation
Capnography
Carboxyhemoglobin
Central venous pressure (CVP)
Flexible fiberoptic bronchoscopy (FFB)
Fluid-balance management
Full-thickness burns
Hyperbaric therapy
Nutritional assessment in weaning
Smoke inhalation
Ventilator weaning

INTRODUCTION

The following case describes parts of the clinical course of Eliza Hayes, a 43-year-old female victim of a house fire. Remember, some data have been withheld from you to facilitate brevity and promote problem solving.

Eliza Hayes was rescued by firefighters after she was found unconscious in her home. Her daughter, who lives in a basement apartment in the building, stated that approximately 25 minutes elapsed from the time she first smelled smoke to the time her mother was rescued. The patient's daughter has suggested that Ms. Hayes might have fallen asleep while smoking. Ms. Hayes was given initial treatment at the scene by firefighters, and she arrived in the EW receiving *bag-valve-mask (BVM) ventilation* with 100% oxygen. Use the clinical notations tables to follow the course of this case.

Clinical Notations: 3:34 AM

General Care	RC Assessments	RC Interventions	Recommendations
Admission, 3:34 AM	43-yr-old female: Approximately 57 kg.	100% oxygen via BVM.	Assess and provide resuscitative
IV (central peripheral) initiated.	Burns over face, head, neck, arms, and part of chest—*full thickness*.	Full assessment. Suctioned gray-black sputum from oropharynx.	measures, and protect and maintain
Ringer's lactate infused (250 mL/h).	Source of burn: House fire.	First RCP continues ventilating with	airway. Ensure

ABGs pending.	May have fallen asleep while smoking.	BVM. Second RCP prepares for FFB.	oxygenation and ventilation.
Electrolytes pending.	Approx. area: 35% of BSA is burned.		
Type and cross pending.	RR = 5 (spontaneous).		
House officer attempted to intubate orally and nasally.	HR = 58. BP = 95/65. SpO$_2$ = 100%. No verbal responses.		
Requested *FFB* to assist with intubation.	Withdraws from painful stimuli and opens eyes. BS reveal few crackles.		

BSA = body surface area, BVM = bag-valve-mask, *FFB = flexible fiberoptic bronchoscopy*.

⇨ Thought Prompts

1. Analyze the initial assessments and evaluate the following for risk factors. (Explain whether there are high, moderate, or low risks associated, and present evidence to support your conclusion.)

Patient's ability to maintain airway patency

Patient's ability to maintain adequate oxygenation

Patient's ability to maintain adequate ventilation

Patient's ability to maintain adequate fluid balance

Patient's risk of infection

2. Describe a monitoring plan for each of the following at-risk systems:

Respiratory:

Cardiovascular:

Renal:

Immune:

Integumentary:

3. Other than fluid administration, what task might be performed via the central venous catheter that has been placed?
4. How may the FFB assist in intubation? Explain the procedure.
5. What other assessments should be performed to evaluate oxygenation?
6. What type of precaution process should be initiated to minimize the risk of infection?
7. Is the use of 100% oxygen justified in this instance? Explain your answer.

Clinical Notations: 4:00 AM

General Care	RC Assessments	RC Interventions	Recom- mendations
4:00 AM NG tube inserted and attached to suction. Urinary catheter inserted. Morphine sulfate administered.	Oral intubation with 7-mm endotracheal tube Labs @ 3:40 AM: ABGs (initial): $PaO_2 = 128$ $PaCO_2 = 50$ pH = 7.10 $HCO_3^- = 18$ *COHb = 50%* K = 6.9 Na = 121 Hgb = 12 WBC = 9000/mm³ Urine output: 35 mL/h HR = 110 *CVP (central venous pressure)* = 5 mm Hg BP = 100/68	Assess tube placement and secure tube. Ventilate via endo- tracheal tube.	Prevent tissue damage when securing airway.

⇨ Thought Prompts

8. Examine the relationship between the oximetry and co-oximetry values and explain why they differ.
9. Given the assessment data in the above table, evaluate Ms. Hayes' fluid status.
10. Describe at least two methods of securing an oral endotracheal tube that would be appropriate in this case. Explain your rationale.
11. Given a barometric pressure of 760 mm Hg, compute the alveolar-arterial oxygen gradient.
12. Compute the arterial oxygen content, as well.
13. Make evaluative statements regarding each of these values (CaO_2 and AaO_2). (Are they normal, slightly deviated from the norm, or critical levels?)
14. Do other forms of intervention exist that may have an impact on Ms. Hayes' oxygenation status?
15. Present the pros and cons of transporting a patient such as Ms. Hayes to a hyperbaric chamber for treatment.
16. Describe *hyperbaric therapy* and explain its desired outcome.

Clinical Notations: 4:00 AM (*Continued*)

General Care	RC Assessments	RC Interventions	Recom- mendations
4:00 AM	*Capnographic* tracing:		

⇨ Thought Prompts

17. Analyze the capnographic data and explain your interpretation.
18. According to the data, has the tube been placed properly?
19. Describe airway care strategies that would reduce the risk of airway trauma in this case.

Clinical Notations: 4:10 AM

General Care	RC Assessments	RC Interventions	Recom- mendations
4:10 AM	ECG observed:		

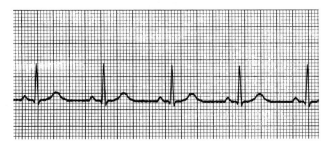

⇨ Thought Prompts

20. Determine the rhythm and rate shown in the above figure.
21. Is any intervention indicated? If so, what?
22. If this rhythm were to continue and symptoms were to worsen, what electrical therapy would be indicated?

Clinical Notations: 4:15 AM to 5:00 AM

General Care	RC Assessments	RC Interventions	Recom- mendations
4:15 AM		MV: $V_t = 0.6$ L $FIO_2 = 1.00$ RR = 12 SIMV Flow rate = 60 L/min Alarms and limits set correctly	Perform system checks q 2 h. Airway and cuff care prn @ least q shift. Obtain sputum sample. Wean from MV per protocol.
5:00 AM	HR = 100 sinus. Occasional spontaneous breaths noted. Responds to verbal stimuli by opening eyes and focusing. Squeezes hand when asked.		

⇨ Thought Prompts

23. What is your evaluation of Eliza Hayes' condition at this point?
24. Determine appropriate objectives for: airway management, oxygenation, ventilation, *fluid balance management,* infection control, and optimal recovery. Then record the RC plan.

Objectives:

Interventions:

Evaluations of outcome:

Clinical Notations: Day 2, 1:30 AM

General Care	RC Assessments	RC Interventions	Recom- mendations
Day 2, 1:30 AM	Bronchospasm noted with wheezing throughout lung fields. Patient coughing frequently. Sinus tachycardia of 140 noted. Thickening of circum- ferential neck and chest eschars noted.		

⇨ Thought Prompts

25. Make recommendations to adjust the RC plan appropriately at this time.
26. How may circumferential eschars affect the patient's spontaneous ventilation ability?

Clinical Notations: Days 3 and 4

General Care	RC Assessments	RC Interventions	Recom- mendations
Day 3, 8:00 AM 12:00 PM 4:00 PM 8:00 PM	Static compliance: 25 mL/cm H_2O 25 23 22	MV settings maintained.	
Day 4, 12:00 AM 4:00 AM 8:00 AM	22 21 20 COHb = 0.5%. ABG is WNL. VS stable. CVP = 8 mm Hg. Urine output = 100 mL/h. WBC = 21,000/mm³. Temp (rectal): 39°C.		

⇨ Thought Prompts

27. Draw conclusion(s) based on the data in the above table.
28. Would you recommend any changes to the RC plan at this point?
29. Could the plan have been regulated at an earlier point to prevent this problem?

30. If the CXR reveals a left lateral lower lobe infiltrate, what postural drainage position would be appropriate?

Clinical Notations: Day 5

General Care	RC Assessments	RC Interventions	Recom- mendations
Day 5	CXR resolving ABGs and labs WNL Urine output = 60 mL/h CVP = 8 mm Hg Spontaneous RR = 6–8 bpm BP = 128/84 HR = 88 K = 3.2 Na = 148 Total protein: 5.2	FIO$_2$ weaned to 35% RR = 10 V$_t$ = 650 mL	

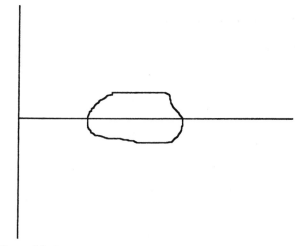

Figure 19–1. Eliza Hayes postextubation pulmonary function test (PFT).

⇨ Thought Prompts

31. What conditions and/or criteria, noted by the assessment data in the Clinical Notations: Day 5, will need to be optimized or corrected before successful *ventilator weaning* may be accomplished?

32. Obtain a copy of the AARC Clinical Practice Guidelines. After consulting the CPGs and seeking further explanations, describe method(s) of *assessing nutritional status* in the critically ill patient.

33. Create a weaning RC plan for Eliza Hayes.

34. Determine criteria that are useful in predicting successful extubation.

35. Analyze the flow-volume loop tracing in Figure 19–1. Determine the likely problem that Eliza Hayes would be demonstrating by such a tracing, performed several days postextubation.

Bibliography

DesJardins, T: Clinical Manifestations and Assessment of Respiratory Disease, ed 3. Mosby-Year Book, St. Louis, 1995.

Farzan, S: A Concise Handbook of Respiratory Disease, ed 3. Appleton & Lange, Stamford, CT, 1992.

Goldenberg Klein, D: Management of persons with burns. In Phipps, W: Medical-Surgical Nursing: Concepts and Clinical Practice, ed 4. Mosby, St. Louis, 1991.

Kacmarek, R and Pierson, D: Foundations of Respiratory Care. Churchill-Livingstone, New York, 1992.

Scanlan, C, Spearman, C and Sheldon, R: Egan's Fundamentals of Respiratory Care, ed 6. Mosby, St. Louis, 1995.

Weaver, LK: Hyperbaric treatment of respiratory emergencies. Respiratory Care 37:720–734, 1992.

Wilkins, RL and Dexter, JR: Respiratory Disease: A Case Study Approach to Patient Care, ed 2. FA Davis, Philadelphia, 1997.

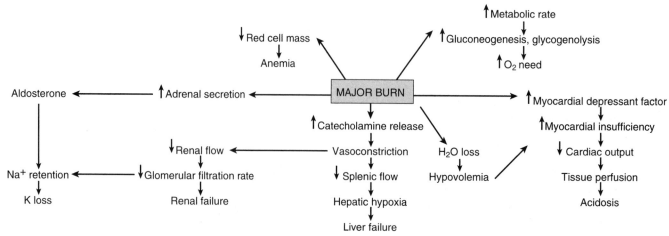

Figure 19–2. Pathophysiology of major burns. (From Goldenberg Klein, D: Management of persons with burns. In Phipps, W: Medical-Surgical Nursing: Concepts and Clinical Practice, ed 4. Mosby-Year Book, St. Louis, 1991, p. 2159, with permission.)

PRACTICE QUESTIONS

1. Fluid status may be evaluated by assessing:
   I. Urine output
   II. Blood pressure
   III. Skin turgor
   IV. Jugular venous distention
   V. Maximum inspiratory pressure
      A. I, II, III, IV, and V
      B. I, III, and V
      C. I, II, III, and IV
      D. I, II, and IV
      E. II and IV

2. Measurement of central venous pressure is most closely reflected by:
   A. Pulmonary capillary wedge pressure
   B. Blood pressure
   C. Systolic pulmonary artery pressure
   D. Right atrial pressure
   E. Pulse pressure

3. Hypokalemia is detected when:
   A. Calcium <45 mEq/dL.
   B. Calcium <3.5 mEq/L.
   C. Potassium <3.5 mEq/L.
   D. Sodium <145 mEq/dL.
   E. Potassium <7.0 mEq/L.

4. If a patient were to contract a nosocomial staphylococcal infection, which of the following is the most likely transmission route?
   A. Improper handwashing
   B. Urinary bladder catheterization
   C. Another patient's coughing
   D. Exchange of body fluids
   E. A dietary source

5. Which of the following descriptives would *not* be interpreted as a sign of chronic airway obstruction?
   A. Stridor
   B. Dyspnea
   C. Decreased FRC
   D. Decreased FEV
   E. Prolonged expiratory time

6. Respiratory distress may occur when carboxyhemoglobin levels reach:
   A. 5 to 10 percent
   B. 10 to 20 percent
   C. 20 to 30 percent
   D. 30 to 40 percent
   E. 40 to 50 percent

7. Given the need to inititate hyperbaric oxygen therapy, the RCP would suggest the use of:
   A. A monoplace chamber
   B. A multiplace chamber
   C. A submariner chamber
   D. A laminar chamber
   E. A or B

8. The most appropriate clinical outcome measurements associated with metabolic calorimetry of a ventilated patient would consist of:
   A. Statistical comparing of like patients
   B. Reversal of present disease state
   C. The measurement of resting energy expenditure
   D. Successful manipulation of the ventilator based on oxygen consumption
   E. Improved pulmonary function

9. An absolute contraindication to the use of postural drainage is:
   A. Intracranial pressure of >15 mm Hg
   B. Hemorrhage with unstable blood pressure
   C. Rib fractures with flail chest
   D. Pulmonary edema
   E. Acute spinal injury

10. Interpret the cardiac rate from the tracing below:
    A. 90
    B. 75
    C. 150
    D. 115
    E. 200

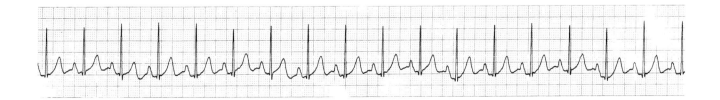

ACTIVITY

Use the following rating scale to evaluate your skill level:

	1 Very High	2 High	3 Fair	4 Low	5 Very Low
1. Level of knowledge regarding care of burn and *smoke inhalation* victims					
2. Level of assessment ability in a case such as that of E. Hayes					
3. Level of planning skill (RC plan)					
4. Level of critical thinking ability as applied to RC					
5. Level of skill in trouble-shooting and problem solving in RC					

Analyze your self-rating and propose goals for your own improvement. How could your expertise in this area be improved? What resources are available to you?

Appendix A
Tips on Taking Clinical Simulation Examinations

There are some obvious points to consider when preparing for the NBRC Clinical Simulation Examination. They include: practice, practice, and more practice. As an educator I see no greater challenge to the individual RCP in regard to credentialing than that of passing the Clinical Simulation Examination. Almost everything in this test is a major challenge: the format, the content, and the required skill level. One cannot underestimate the advantage of working in environments that foster the skill of critical thinking. Using commercially provided clinical simulations (in particular, the Self-Assessment Examination from Applied Measurement Professionals, Inc.), completing case study work (in particular this book, of course), and participating in supervised clinical practice opportunities allow you to apply the skills you will need for competent performance.

In addition to this general advice, the following excerpt from D. Theron VanHooser proves quite insightful:

The Clinical Simulation Examination: Do's & Don'ts

Purpose of the Patient Management Problem
- Gather appropriate clinical data
- Interpret and/or synthesize data
- Solve problems
- Make clinical judgments and/or decisions

The three components:

Components	Function
Scenario	Provide a short, descriptive paragraph which begins the simulation and sets the stage for the patient management problem-solving process. The scenario contains three important pieces of information: 1. Physical Setting 2. Information about the patient 3. Practitioner's role and task in the problem.
Information gathering (IG)	Assess candidate's ability to gather appropriate clinical data including physical and laboratory assessment in order to evaluate a patient and make decisions relative to patient care.
Decision Making	Designed to test the candidate's ability to interpret and/or synthesize data in order to solve problems and/or make decisions.

Scenario:

Do	Do Not
Do read the scenario carefully before selecting responses in any section.	Do not make assumptions about the scenario; you should not try to guess or anticipate what is expected or "read" anything into the problem that is not presented.
Do identify the three aspects of the scenario.	Do not become distracted if the scenario presents a situation in which you have never been (e.g., the ER physician at your hospital has never asked for your recommendations, and yet you are being asked to assist in a patient assessment and provide advice). Rely upon your knowledge and experience; try to imagine yourself in the situation and make decisions consistent with good patient care.

Scenario *Continued*

Do	**Do Not**
Do use a pencil to mark the important information you may need to refer to later in decision making. Notations may be made in the margins of the test booklet.	Do not read ahead to attempt to determine what will evolve in the problem. The problem sections are scrambled and have various branches, so it is not meaningful to read ahead.

Information Gathering:

Do   **Do Not**

Selecting information

Do consider all options and use a pencil to lightly mark each option you wish to select before developing the responses.	Do not be curious about new or unusual terms. If you are unfamiliar with what an option presents, you probably should not select it; the information may not be helpful if it is new to you and you do not understand it.
Do select all options which will provide meaningful information; you will not be rewarded for selecting minimal data.	Do not select all options. Some of the information may be too time consuming, costly, irrelevant, or inappropriate. As in actual practice, some information is unnecessary and wasteful; you will be penalized for selecting such information.

Analyzing the information

Do decide which information will be the most helpful in analyzing the patient's situation; be sure to pay attention to that information which is most helpful to your analysis.	Do not misread the data. Use care and precision to read and analyze the responses. Do not assume things which are not printed and be careful not to transpose numbers.
Do form a mental image of the patient and the situation as it would be in your hospital or clinic. This will help you decide what to do next.	
Do decide if the situation is an emergency or not, and select responses appropriately. Selecting tests or procedures which delay care in an emergency setting will result in a lower score.	
Do decide if the information selected is complete and review the remaining options to see if you may have overlooked any which will provide appropriate information to confirm your analysis of the findings.	

Decision Making:

Do	**Do Not**
Do read all the options carefully and determine the most appropriate actions to take, based upon the information you gained from previous sections and the patient's present condition.	Do not be distressed if your favorite mode of therapy is missing from the options. Just as in actual clinical practice, there is more than one way to achieve the therapeutic goal. Of the options presented, choose the best for managing the patient in a safe, effective manner.
Do think about your choice before uncovering the response. Unlike a multiple-choice test, you cannot change your mind and erase. Once a response is uncovered, you will have to deal with the outcome of the decision you have made.	Do not uncover another response in a "Choose only one section," unless directed to do so. The majority of the decision-making sections will be the "choose only one" type and you must follow the response instructions exactly, even if you realize you should have selected another response. However, some decision-making sections require multiple decisions where you are instructed to select as many as you feel are indicated.

Do read the response carefully. Take your time and make sure you understand the instructions or results in the response. "Physician disagrees" may or may not indicate incorrect response. In an actual clinical setting, physicians may not always agree with your recommended mode of therapy.

Do keep a written map of the sections as you proceed through the problem. This will help you go back to check previous blood gases, etc. Use your pencil and write down the section letters in the order in which you encounter them in the margin or inside cover of your test booklet.

Do not select therapeutics with which you are not familiar. You may lose points for choosing incorrectly; and if you are unfamiliar with the therapy, it stands to reason that you may not be able to apply it correctly.

Do not read ahead in the problem. The feedback in the response will give you the facts you need to proceed. Do not attempt to find out more information by reading scenarios in other sections. The sections are scrambled, so the information may not be current or pertinent. Do not make any assumptions about care of the patient for which supporting information is not provided.

To further acquaint yourself with the content of the NBRC Clinical Simulation Examination, you should acquire a copy of the NBRC Study Guide or other commercially available guides.

Appendix B
Troubleshooting Tips: A Troubleshooting Chart

Note the essential structure of the process of troubleshooting

Identify the Problem
(gather information; respond to signal for help; consider routine or common occurrences;
rule out other problems; guess and check)

Isolate the Problem
(separate equipment from patient; perform tests; follow safety
procedures; remove problem)

Remediate/Repair/Resolve/Regulate
(perform corrective actions . . . assure safety)

Evaluate Troubleshooting Outcome/Prevent Future Occurrence
(assure problem is corrected/consider policy or procedure changes)

Document/Report/Determine Follow-Up Plan, If Needed
(record all pertinent data; file appropriately; communicate to involved parties)

It is often helpful in any troubleshooting situation to make "if/then" statements. For instance, when troubleshooting a ventilator low pressure alarm condition, state to yourself: *If* there is drop in the system pressure, *then* there could be a leak in the system. Assumptions like these will likely steer you in the right direction to troubleshoot the problem.

Appendix C
Common Equations Used throughout the Text

Estimated tidal volume:

$VT_{mechanical} = \text{IBW} \times 10\text{–}15 \text{ mL/kg}$

(Note that values < 10 mL/kg are used when indicated, as in permissive hypercapnea)

Calculating inspiratory time:

$IT = \dfrac{\text{TCT}}{\text{I} + \text{E}}$

(Where TCT is total cycle time and I & E are symbols for inspiratory-expiratory ratio)

Changing minute ventilation:

$\text{Desired } \dot{V}E = \dfrac{\dot{V}E \text{ known} \times \text{Pa}CO_2}{\text{desired Pa}CO_2}$

Compliance:

$C_{dynamic} = \dfrac{V_t}{P_{peak} - \text{PEEP}}$

$C_{static} = \dfrac{V_t}{P_{plateau} - \text{PEEP}}$

$R_{airway} = \dfrac{P_{peak} - P_{plateau}}{\dot{V}}$

(Where $\dot{V}$ is flow)

Dead space to tidal volume ratio:

$VD/V_t = \dfrac{\text{Pa}CO_2 - \text{P}ECO_2}{\text{Pa}CO_2}$

(Where $\text{P}ECO_2$ is expired carbon dioxide pressure)

Alveolar oxygen:

$PAO_2 = (\text{P}B - \text{P}H_2O) - \text{Pa}CO_2/.8$
$AaO_2 = PAO_2 - PaO_2$

(Where PB is barometric pressure)
(The gradient between alveolar and arterial oxygen pressures)

Cardiac output:

$\dot{Q} = \dfrac{\dot{V}O_2}{(C_{a-v}O_2) \times 10}$

(Where $\dot{V}O_2$ is oxygen consumption and $C_{a-v}O_2$ is the difference between arterial oxygen content and mixed venous oxygen content)

Estimation of shunt:

$\dot{Q}s/\dot{Q}T = \dfrac{AaO_2 \times .003}{(C_{a-v}O_2) + (AaO_2 \times .003)}$

Oxygen duration (cylinder) calculations:

$\text{Compressed gas duration} = \dfrac{\text{tank factor} \times \text{PSI}}{\text{flow (in liters)}}$

(Where PSI is pressure within the tank and the common tank factors 3.14 for H cylinders and .28 for E cylinders)

$\text{Liquid oxygen duration} = \dfrac{\text{content of cylinder}}{\text{liter flow}}$

Appendix D
Glasgow Coma Scale

I. Best Motor Response

Obeys	6
Localizes	5
Withdraws (flexion)	4
Abnormal flexion	3
Extensor response	2
No response	1

II. Verbal Response

Oriented	5
Confused conversation	4
Inappropriate words	3
Incomprehensible sounds	2
No verbal response	1

III. Eye Opening

Spontaneous	4
To speech	3
To pain	2
None	1

COMA SCORE = I + II + III
(Max: 15   Lowest: 3)

Answers to Practice Questions

CHAPTER 1

1. E PBL has become an important part of organizations worldwide and is based on the presentation of problems to learners.
2. A Concept maps do not necessarily reveal cause-and-effect information.
3. B Structured lectures are not basic components of PBL but may be part of the overall teaching strategy.
4. B All other statements are positive statements regarding PBL.
5. C Basic recall of information is not a critical thinking function.
6. C No resources support the statement.
7. D Recall, application, and analysis are the basic categories of the NBRC written examinations.
8. E All are true.
9. D Cause-and-effect diagrams represent linear illustrations of causal relationships between information.
10. A Group discussion, guided inquiry, and independent study are all components of PBL.

CHAPTER 2

1. E All are essential to developing CT.
2. B Memorization is not in itself a CT skill—all others are (see Table 2–1).
3. E All are important in good decision making.
4. D Estimating, assuming, and grasping principles are functions of CT, whereas believing and preferring are subjective responses (and not based on objective evidence).
5. A All others are strategies for practicing CT; only A assesses it.
6. C Metacognition, the thinking about one's thinking, is prompted by allowing an incubation period.
7. A This activity is not necessarily a consensus-seeking activity but, rather, is focused toward multiple-perspective viewing and logic-based argument.
8. B Reliance on memorized data is a tactic more likely associated with the novice.
9. C Having a busy workday is a stimulating experience, likely to prompt some problem solving, while A, B, D, and E are situations in which emotion and, therefore, subjectivity may dominate the thinking.

CHAPTER 3

1. E Judgment formation is the essence of the evaluation process.

2. D ABGs and capnography are not cost-efficient tools for a limited assessment.
3. E All represent good sources of this information.
4. D Evidence is produced through assessment. A, B, and D are outcomes. C; although documentation is critical, it is the tool for recording assessments; it is not the actual assessment.
5. A All other assessments are unusual events for the given population.
6. E Invasive procedures should *not* be performed unless clearly needed to improve patient outcome.
7. B This is the correct order.
8. C CT is the essential ingredient in RC assessment.
9. C Although assessment may be focused on any of the choices, it is best defined by C.

CHAPTER 4

1. B Judgment formation *is* evaluation. It is the outcome of the process and therefore not a *component* of it.
2. C Preliminary results have not been tested over time, and they do not represent a broad scope. They do not represent a model for comparison.
3. D *Measurement* validity refers to measuring the intended subject.
4. B *Reliability* refers to consistency or repeatability.
5. A B, satisfaction, and C, the therapeutic process, are targets of impact evaluation. D, goal attainment, is the target of outcome evaluation.
6. B A, compliance with standards, and C, RCP performance, are process measures. D, goal attainment, is an outcome evaluation measure.
7. D A and C are process measures. B is an impact target.
8. D Decreasing departmental costs do not define an overall evaluation, although cost-saving measures may be discovered as a by-product of the evaluation process.

CHAPTER 5

1. Indications for RC modalities:
   A Tracheostomy tube in place, bypassing upper airway.
   B Production of large amounts of sputum 25–30 mL/day with poor cough ability.
2. A Bland aerosol therapy—continuous/heated.
   B Postural drainage—q 6 h or to be determined by outcome of therapy.
3. A Bland aerosol therapy—to minimize humidity deficit, related to bypassed upper airway.
   B Postural drainage—to mobilize secretions and decrease retention of sputum (production decrease to <25 mL/day) to promote clear breath sounds.

4. Monitor by: observation/physical examination.
    auscultation.

5. A The objective of minimizing humidity deficit will be evaluated by lack of further secretion retention, as evidenced by auscultation, CXR, and sputum production.

    B The objective of mobilizing secretions will be measured by observation of decrease in sputum production to <25 mL/day, clear breath sounds, and CXR also.

6. Negative events associated with aerosol therapy may include: wheezing or bronchospasm, bronchoconstriction, infection, overhydration, and patient discomfort.

    Other indications for changing therapy may include worsening ventilatory state and the need for mechanical ventilation (Refer to the AARC clinical practice guideline on bland aerosol administration.)

    Negative events associated with postural drainage include: hypoxemia, increased intracranial pressure, acute hypotension, pulmonary hemorrhage, pain or injury, vomiting and aspiration, bronchospasm, and dysrythmia.

    Positive events that warrant modification to the plan could include: patient progress including extubation and/or achievement of the set therapeutic objectives.

7. The plan should be reevaluated every 24 to 72 hours or when a change in patient status indicates the need for reevaluation.

8. The RC plan:

    Indications: tracheostomy tube in place, bypassing upper airway.
    production of large amounts of sputum 25–30 mL/day with poor cough ability.

    Objectives: bland aerosol—to minimize humidity deficit, related to bypassed upper airway.

    Postural drainage—to mobilize secretions and decrease retention of sputum (production decrease to <25 mL/day) to promote clear breath sounds.

    Interventions: A Bland aerosol therapy—continuous.
    B Postural drainage—q 6 h or to be determined by outcome of therapy.

    Evaluations: A The objective of minimizing humidity deficit will be evaluated by lack of further secretion retention, as evidenced by auscultation, observation of CXR, and sputum production.
    B The objective of mobilizing secretions will be measured by observation of decrease in sputum production to <25 mL/day, clear breath sounds, and CXR also.

9. Transport this patient, using a heat moisture exchanger. Monitor by physical observation, vital signs, and pulse oximetry, as well as by subjective patient communications.

10. If the patient's oxygen demand increased, the F_{IO_2} would need to be increased, and further assessments would follow.

    If the patient were to experience respiratory failure, the likely therapeutic intervention would include positive pressure ventilation and close monitoring.

CHAPTER 6

1. D Although all are important, the best place to start a time management program is with a time analysis of the current situation.

2. C Although time management may improve efficiency, the two terms are not synonymous. Time management programs are instituted for numerous reasons.

3. A Clinical competence would be assessed through other evaluative means but not directly through a time analysis.

4. B Although all of these negative events may occur, the lack of time structure would be the initial problem.

5. D Carefully chosen equipment storage would contribute to the efficiency of an organization by allowing for time savings in equipment gathering. This may in turn relate to effectiveness, but first and foremost is efficiency. All other choices (A, B, C, and E) would need to be equally effective and efficient.

6. A Sometimes the long-range priorities must be attended to without the interference of short-time tasks.

7. C See Table 6–2.

8. B Changing the daily schedule would resolve or prevent time conflict, while all the other choices are examples of time conflict.

9. C

10. A

11. B

CHAPTER 7

1. E Refer to the AARC Clinical Practice Guidelines.

2. B The maximal inspiration.

3. D Hypoxemia may result from or occur in tandem with atelectasis but does not necessarily produce it.

4. C Refer to the AARC Clinical Practice Guidelines.

5. E Refer to the AARC Clinical Practice Guidelines.

6. E All are signs of atelectasis.

7. B Objectives for oxygen therapy include maintaining normoxia, decreasing myocardial work, and providing O_2 for postoperative patients, *but* oxygen will stabilize acid-base balance. And premature infants would not routinely be oxygenated with PaO_2 or 90 to 100 mm Hg. Their safe range is 50 to 80 mm Hg.

8. A The objective datum of clear CXR is the optimal response, as this is one indication for incentive spirometry.

9. C Demonstration is the most reliable indicator.

10. A Refer to the AARC Clinical Practice Guidelines.

CHAPTER 8

1. C

2. B

3. D

4. A
5. A
6. E
7. A
8. A
9. A
10. E
11. B

CHAPTER 9

1. C
2. B
3. A
4. D
5. D
6. C
7. C
8. A
9. E
10. A

CHAPTER 10

1. B
2. C
3. D
4. D
5. C
6. B
7. D
8. A
9. A
10. B

CHAPTER 11

1. E
2. A
3. C   Refer to applicable CPG.
4. D   Refer to applicable CPG.
5. D   Refer to applicable CPG.
6. A   Refer to applicable CPG.
7. C
8. A

CHAPTER 12

1. C
2. D
3. A
4. A   Intubation not *usually* indicated in LTB.
5. A
6. D
7. B

CHAPTER 13

1. B
2. D
3. C
4. C
5. A
6. C
7. C
8. A
9. B

CHAPTER 14

1. C
2. C
3. A
4. B
5. A
6. C
7. E
8. D
9. A
10. B

CHAPTER 15

1. B and D
2. C
3. B
4. D
5. B
6. B
7. A
8. A
9. A
10. D

CHAPTER 16

1. D
2. B
3. A
4. D
5. E
6. A
7. B
8. E
9. D
10. A

CHAPTER 17

1. E
2. B
3. E
4. A
5. E

6. D
7. B
8. A
9. D
10. A

CHAPTER 18

1. C
2. E
3. B
4. E
5. C
6. B
7. B
8. A

9. D
10. D

CHAPTER 19

1. C
2. D
3. C
4. A
5. C
6. A
7. E
8. D
9. E
10. A

Index

A number followed by an "f" indicates a figure; a number followed by a "t" indicates a table.